UPDATED FOR 2000

Electrotherapeutic Terminology in Physical Therapy

Section on Clinical Electrophysiology

D1525668

American Physical Therapy Association

Contents

Contributors 5

Introduction 6

I. Electrophysics: Basic Terminology 7

II. Types and Characteristics of Therapeutic Currents 10
  A. General Observations 10
  B. Types of Currents 12
    1. Direct Current 12
      a. Descriptive characteristics of DC 12
      b. Time-dependent characteristics of DC 12
      c. Amplitude-dependent characteristics of DC 12
        1) Amplitude 12
        2) Peak amplitude 13
        3) Root mean square amplitude 13
      d. Modulation of DC 13
        1) Amplitude modulations 13
          a) Reversing DC 13
          b) Ramped DC 13
        2) Timing modulations 13
          a) Interrupted DC 13
            i) ON time 13
            ii) OFF time 14

    2. Alternating Current 14
      a. Descriptive characteristics of AC 14
        1) Waveform 14
        2) Symmetric and asymmetric cycles (waveforms) 15
        3) Balanced vs unbalanced cycles (waveforms) 15
      b. Time-dependent characteristics of AC 15
        1) Classification of AC 15
        2) Frequency 15
        3) Rise and decay times 15
        4) Period 16
      c. Amplitude-dependent characteristics of AC 16
        1) Amplitude 16
          a) Peak amplitude 16
          b) Root mean square amplitude 16
      d. Time- and amplitude-dependent characteristics of AC 17
        1) Phase charge 17
        2) Cycle charge 17
      e. Modulation of AC 17
        1) Amplitude modulations 17
          a) Ramped AC 18

2) Time modulations 19
   a) Burst 19
     i) Burst duration 19
     ii) Interburst interval 19
   b) Interrupted AC 19
     i) ON time 20
     ii) OFF time 20
3. Pulsed or Pulsatile Current 20
  a. Descriptive characteristics of PC 20
   1) Waveform 21
   2) Phase 21
    a) Monophasic 21
    b) Biphasic 21
   3) Symmetric and asymmetric waveforms 22
   4) Balanced vs unbalanced waveforms 22
  b. Time-dependent characteristics of PC 22
   1) Rise and decay times 22
   2) Phase duration 23
   3) Pulse duration 23
   4) Interphase interval 23
   5) Interpulse interval 24
   6) Frequency 24
   7) Period 24
  c. Amplitude-dependent characteristics of PC 24
   1) Amplitude 24
    a) Peak amplitude 25
    b) Root mean square amplitude 25
  d. Time- and amplitude-dependent characteristics of PC 25
   1) Phase charge 25
   2) Pulse charge 25
  e. Modulations of PC 25
   1) Amplitude modulations 25
    a) Ramped PC 25
    b) Reversing PC 26
   2) Timing modulations 27
    a) Phase- or pulse-duration modulations 27
    b) Burst 27
     i) Burst duration 27
     ii) Interburst interval 27
    c) Interrupted PC 27
     i) ON time 27
     ii) OFF time 28
   3) Frequency modulations 30
    a) Pulse-frequency (-rate) modulation 30
    b) Burst-frequency modulation 30

References-Therapeutic Currents **31**

III. Instrumentation Design and Application Considerations **32**
  A. Constant Current and Voltage Stimulators 32
    1. Constant (or regulated) current instruments 32
    2. Constant (or regulated) voltage instruments 32
  B. Stimulation Electrodes 32
    1. Types of electrodes 32
    2. Electrode coupling media 33
    3. Relationship between electrode surface area and current 33
    4. Electrode configurations 33
      a. Description of electrode placement 34
        1) Monopolar 34
        2) Bipolar 34
        3) Quadripolar 34
      b. Ground electrode 35
  C. Description of Electrical Stimulation Applications 35
    1. Clinical applications of electrotherapeutic currents 36
      a. Pain Management 36
      b. Neuromuscular Dysfunction 36
        1) Innervated muscle 36
        2) Denervated muscle 36
      c. Joint Mobility 36
      d. Tissue Repair 36
      e. Acute and Chronic Edema (Swelling) 37
      f. Peripheral Blood Flow 37
      g. Urine and Fecal Incontinence 37
      h. Iontophoresis 37
    2. Vague terms 37
      a. Trade or brand names 37
      b. Characteristics of current 37
        1) Waveform or current specifications 37
        2) Relative amplitude specifications 38
        3) Frequency specifications 38
        4) Duty cycle specifications 39
      c. Techniques 39

Appendix 40
References 45

Committee Members:

Gad Alon, PT, PhD, Chair
Andrew J Robinson, PT, PhD
Neil Spielholz, PT, PhD
Luther Kloth, PT, MS
David Selkowitz, PT, MS
Meryl Gersh, PT, MS
Lucinda L Baker, PT, PhD

Consultant:

J Patrick Reilly, PhD
(Emeritus)
The Johns Hopkins University
Applied Physics Laboratory

The committee also recognizes the input of several members of the Section on Clinical Electrophysiology of the American Physical Therapy Association in the early phase of writing this document.

INTRODUCTION

In 1986, the Section on Clinical Electrophysiology of the American Physical Therapy Association formed an ad hoc committee of clinicians, educators, and researchers to address the issue of the use of undefined and misleading terms and units in electrotherapy. The committee's major concern was that treatment applications of electrotherapy can be neither understood clearly nor replicated because of 1) incomplete specification of stimulator output characteristics and clinical application procedures, and 2) lack of standardization of terminology among the disciplines involved in electrotherapy. An additional concern has been the realization that in the absence of evidence-based terminology, clinicians, educators, and researchers alike are adding to the confusion. The committee developed the "Electrotherapeutic Terminology" monograph to clarify terminology and foster uniformity of communication in product development and performance, clinical and research applications, and publications.

The success of the original document inspired the Section on Clinical Electrophysiology to appoint a new ad hoc committee consisting of a few of the original members and few new members to revise and update the monograph. By using the information provided in this new edition, clinicians and researchers should be able to communicate more effectively the details of procedures and results of their use of electrotherapy exclusive of the thermal effects of electrical currents. The manufacturers of electrotherapeutic devices should be able to convey accurate and concise information to clinicians about output characteristics of their equipment. Other groups, including physicians and biomedical engineers, may find this publication useful in enhancing communication across professions. As technological changes and advances occur, periodic revisions of this monograph will be made.

This monograph does not provide clinical procedures or rationale for therapeutic applications of electrical currents. References from peer-reviewed publications are cited as examples and are not intended to represent an exhaustive bibliography. Similarly, the figures throughout the document are intended to enhance understanding of the terminology rather than illustrate all possible electrical current configurations to which the terms may apply. This monograph is not conceived to limit the development or advancement of electrotherapeutic interventions or scientific inquiry. Rather, it provides evidenced-based terminology for existing electrotherapeutic products and applications.

For ease of use, this publication has been styled in outline form and focuses on standardization of the terminology of three areas:

I. Basic Terminology in Electrophysics
II. Types and Characteristics of Therapeutic Currents
III. Instrumentation Design and Application Considerations

The American Physical Therapy Association, together with the Section on Clinical Electrophysiology, presents this document with the hope and expectation that it will further enhance communication and collaboration among clinicians, researchers, academicians, and manufacturers of electrotherapeutic devices.

I. Electrophysics: Basic Terminology

A. _Charge (Q)_: Electrical charge is a fundamental property of matter. Matter either has no net charge (ie, electrically neutral) or is negatively or positively charged. The fundamental particle of negative charge is the electron (e-). An electrically neutral body can become "charged" by either gaining or losing one or more electrons. An electrically neutral substance that gains one or more electrons becomes negatively charged (-), while an electrically neutral substance that loses one or more electrons becomes positively charged (+).

1. Charge is measured in units called _coulombs_, which are specific quantities of electrons (e-). One coulomb contains 6.28×10^{18} electrons. Since an electron is a negatively charged particle, one electron carries a negative charge (Q) of 1.6×10^{-19} coulombs.

2. Charge density is a measure of the electrical charge per unit of an electrode's cross-sectional area. Charge density is expressed as Q/cm^2. However, since the magnitudes of charge typically used in clinical practice are relatively small, charge densities are more likely to be expressed as $\mu Q/cm^2$.

B. _Polarity_: Polarity is the property of having two oppositely charged conductors—one positive, the other negative. In a conductor, free electrons flow from an area containing an excess of electrons (negative polarity) to an area deficient in them (positive polarity).

1. _Cathode_ is the negatively charged pole (or the electron source) of an electrical circuit.

2. _Anode_ is the positively charged pole (or the electron sink) of an electrical circuit.

C. _Voltage (V) (electromotive force [E or EMF])_: The electrical force capable of moving electrons or other charged particles, such as ions, through a conductor between two regions or points is the voltage, which also is known as the potential difference between two points. The voltage between two points is due to the separation of charges between these two points—one region has an excess of electrons compared with the other. These two points, or regions, are "polarized" with respect to one another, so that one is negative and the other is positive.

D. _Current (I)_: The rate of flow of charged particles (electrons or ions) past a specific point in a specific direction is the current. Current is produced in a conductor by the voltage or potential difference between points in a circuit. Current is measured in units of amperes (A) and is defined mathematically as I=Q/t, where I=amperes; Q=coulombs; and t=time (in seconds). If the current in a circuit is 1 amp, 1 coulomb of electrons flows in that circuit each second. In other words, an ampere is a measure of how many electrons are flowing per unit time. In the therapeutic use of electricity, the current that flows in tissues is carried by ions, not by free electrons. In this situation, positively charged ions, such as Na^+, K^+, or H^+, migrate toward the cathode, while negatively charged ions, such as Cl^-, HCO_3^-, and P^- (large protein molecules that are negatively charged) migrate toward the anode.

Note: Since positively charged ions migrate toward the cathode, these ions are known also as cations (ie, attracted to the cathode). Conversely, anions are negatively charged ions that are attracted to the anode.

E. *Power (P)*: Measured in watts (W), power is the time rate of transforming or transferring electrical energy. Power is calculated by multiplying a circuit's voltage (V) times its current (I), or W=VI. And since V=IR, we can also write $W=I^2R$.

F. *Energy (U)*: Energy is the quantity that describes the amount of work done or the potential to do work or create heat. In an electrical circuit, energy is given by the product of power (P or W) and time (t). Expressions for energy can be stated as: U=VIt or U=I2 Rt. Energy is measured in joules (J).

G. *Resistance (R)*: Measured in ohms (Ω), resistance is a property of a conductor that characterizes its opposition to the flow of charged particles. A conductor's resistance is directly proportional to its resistivity rho(Δ) and its length (l), and inversely proportional to its cross-sectional area (A). Resistance typically decreases as the conductor's temperature increases. A conductor's resistance is 1 ohm if a potential difference of 1 volt causes 1 amp to flow through it. This is one form of Ohm's Law, which states R=V/I. Resistance of a wire is independent of frequency, but in biological conductors resistance may increase as frequency decreases (see I and K below).

H. *Conductance (g)*: The inverse of resistance is conductance, which expresses the ease with which charged particles flow through a conductor. Mathematically, conductance is the reciprocal of the conductor's resistance (ie, g=1/R) and is measured in siemens (formerly "mhos"). In other words, high resistance indicates low conductance, and low resistance indicates high conductance.

I. *Ohm's Law*: This is the mathematical expression of how the three properties of voltage, current, and resistance relate to one another. One example of this relationship was given above (R=V/I). Given any two of these properties, the third can be calculated by simple algebraic rearrangement.

J. *Capacitance (C)*: Measured in farads (f), capacitance is the ability of two closely spaced plates to store charge. If one coulomb of charge is stored on the plates of a capacitor when the voltage difference between them is 1 volt, its capacitance is 1 F. Mathematically, this is F=Q/V. A farad is actually a very large amount of charge. In most biological and electronic situations, the charges stored are much smaller, and measured in µF ($1x10^{-6}$F). Since a capacitor is part of a circuit, it contributes to the overall resistance of that circuit. This resistance, sometimes referred to as "capacitative reactance," is inversely related to the frequency of the current (or to the individual pulse durations). Therefore, direct current, which has no frequency (or an infinite pulse duration), meets the highest resistance of the capacitor. As frequency increases (or pulse duration decreases), the capacitor offers less and less resistance to the flow of current. In addition, capacitors affect, in mathematically predictable ways, the time-course with which currents (or voltages) rise and fall within a circuit. Currents passing through biological tissues meet both classical resistance and capacitive reactance. Indeed, much of the membrane physiology depends on the capacitive aspect of these structures.

K. *Inductance (L)*: Expressed as henrys (H), inductance is a measure of the degree to which a varying (alternating) current can induce an electromotive force (V) opposite to the voltage generating the original current. This is known as *inductive reactance*. The inductance in a circuit is 1H if 1V is induced in that circuit when the current changes at a rate of 1A/s. Unlike capacitance, inductance is negligible in biological systems.

L. *Impedance (Z)*: Impedance refers to the resistance in a circuit containing classical resistance in addition to one or both of the frequency-dependent oppositions to current flow mentioned above (ie, capacitive reactance and inductive reactance). Like resistance, impedance is expressed in ohms, but given the symbol Z to distinguish it from simple resistance (R). For biological systems, impedance describes the ratio of voltage to current more accurately than does resistance because impedance is a frequency-dependent measure that includes the effects of capacitive reactance, inductive reactance, and resistance. Because inductive reactance is negligible in biological systems, it can be ignored in determining impedance.

M. *Reactance (X)*: This is a general term applied to the opposition to current flow produced by capacitance (C) or inductance (L) in a circuit. In biological systems, the frequency-dependent component of impedance is primarily due to capacitance.

Reference:

Jay F, ed: IEEE, *Standard Dictionary of Electrical and Electronic Terms*, 2nd ed. New York, NY: IEEE Inc and Wiley-Interscience; 1977.

II. Characteristics of Therapeutic Currents

A. General Observations

1. The distinctions made below between direct current (DC), alternating current (AC), and pulsed current (PC) have been developed to define the types of therapeutic currents used in clinical practice. Our adoption of the term "pulsed current" is not meant to imply a third family of basic currents (there are still only two, direct and alternating), but to give more meaningful descriptions to the "pulsed" waveforms that are actually delivered by the majority of electrotherapeutic devices used by clinicians.

2. Electrotherapeutic currents can be described in both qualitative and quantitative terms. Discussion of currents in qualitative terms only is not recommended. Rather, in written and oral discussions of therapeutic currents, standardized qualitative descriptions and quantitative parameters both should be used to provide a clear and unambiguous understanding of the therapeutic intervention. Illustrations of the current and voltage waveforms as a function of time should accompany qualitative descriptions. The need to describe current and voltage waveforms emerges from the fact that they may not exhibit the same waveform or shape.

3. A recommended system for combining qualitative descriptive terms in the standardized naming of electrotherapeutic currents is offered. The flow chart serves as a guide for combining qualitative characteristics of medical currents to arrive at a consistent description of any particular electro-medical current (**Fig 1**). Furthermore each type of current can be delivered with or without modulations. Current modulations typically are classified as time-modulated or amplitude-modulated, or both (**Fig 2**).

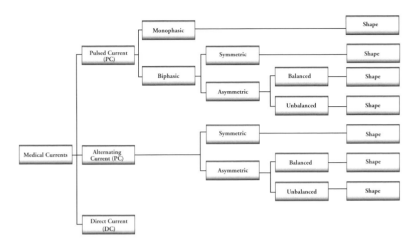

Figure 1
Schematic organization of medical currents and the descriptive terms used to characterize these currents.

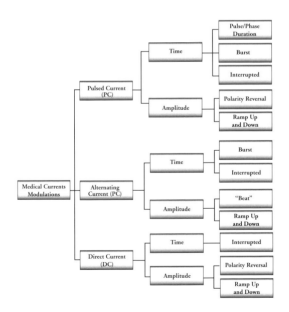

Figure 2
Schematic organization of the systematic modulation in one or more of the amplitude- or time-dependent characteristics of the three medical currents.

B. Types of Currents

1. **Direct Current (DC)** is the continuous unidirectional flow of charged particles. The direction of flow is determined by the polarity selected, with positively charged particles (cations) moving toward the negative pole (cathode) and the negatively charged particles (anions) moving toward the positive pole (anode).

   a. Descriptive characteristics of DC

      1) As defined, DC has no pulses and, therefore, has no waveform associated with it.

   b. Time-dependent characteristics of DC

      1) To be classified as DC for clinical purposes, the flow of charges must continue uninterrupted for at least 1 second.

   c. Amplitude-dependent characteristics of DC

      1) *Amplitude* is the measure of the magnitude of current (or voltage) with reference to the isoelectric (zero) line. Whenever possible, the current and the voltage both should be specified.

      Note: The term "intensity" frequently is used interchangeably with "amplitude." To avoid confusion and inconsistency, the term "intensity" should never be used to describe current or voltage amplitude.

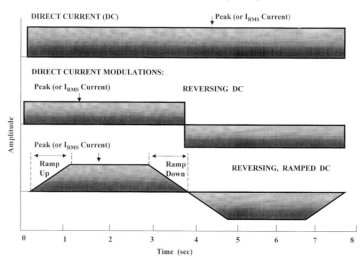

Figure 3

Amplitude-dependent modulations of direct current (DC). Upper graph, Unmodulated, (continuous) DC. Middle graph, Reversing DC. Lower graph, Reversing, ramped DC. The values of peak and I_{RMS} currents are the same in DC. Note that the time scale is expressed in seconds.

2) *Peak amplitude* is the highest amplitude of the current or voltage (**Fig 3**).

3) *Root mean square (RMS) amplitude* represents the current (I_{RMS}) or voltage (V_{RMS}) applied over a specified length of time. The recommended time is 1 second. In DC, peak current and I_{RMS} current amplitudes are the same (**Fig 3**).

d. Modulation of DC
Note: One or more of these modulations may occur simultaneously.

1) *Amplitude modulations* are variations in amplitude over time. The modulations may be sequential or variable.

   a) *Reversing DC* is the reversal of polarity (crossing the isoelectric line) after one second or longer (**Fig 3**).

   b) *Ramped DC* is the gradual increase from and decrease to the isoelectric line of the DC amplitude over 1 second or longer (**Fig 3**).

2) *Timing modulations* are variations in the delivery pattern of the direct current.

   a) *Interrupted DC* means a direct current intermittently ceases to flow for 1 second or longer. The DC, when interrupted, yields ON and OFF times.

     i) *ON time* is the time, typically measured in seconds, during which the DC is delivered in a therapeutic application.

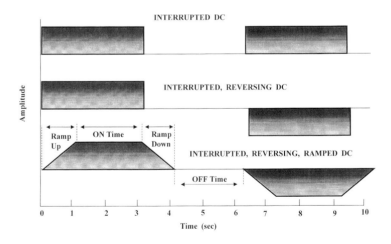

Figure 4
Time-dependent modulation of direct current (DC). Upper graph, Interrupted DC. Middle graph, Interrupted, reversing DC. Lower graph, Interrupted, reversing, ramped DC.

ii) *OFF time* is the time during which DC is not flowing (typically measured in seconds). Interrupted DC, alone and in combination with polarity reversal and ramping, is illustrated in **Fig 4**.

Note: The term "ON time" occasionally includes the ramp-up and ramp-down times and occasionally is exclusive of ramp times. To avoid confusion and inconsistency, the ramp-up and ramp-down times should be specified independently of the ON time. Likewise, the ON time should not include ramp-up or ramp-down times.

2. **Alternating Current (AC)** is the continuous bidirectional flow of charged particles. The change in direction of flow occurs at least once every second.

  a. Descriptive characteristics of AC

    1) *Waveform* is the visual representation of the current or voltage, on the amplitude-time plot. An AC waveform is represented by one cycle. Cycle describes an electrical event that begins when the current (or voltage) departs from the isoelectric line in one direction then crosses the same baseline in the opposite direction. The cycle ends when the current returns again to the baseline. The cycle can be divided into two halves: The first half cycle ends when the current crosses the baseline the first time; the second half ends when the current returns to the baseline the second time. Each half cycle is considered one phase. The waveforms of the cycle phases often are described by their geometric shape (rectangular, sinusoidal, triangular, etc) (**Fig 5**).

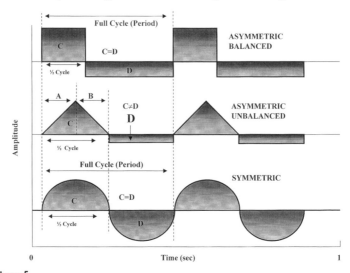

Figure 5
Examples of alternating current of different shapes. A=rise time, B=fall time, C=area under the curve representing electrical charge of the first half cycle, and D=charge of the second half cycle. If C=D, the cycle's electrical charge is balanced. If C≠D, the cycle's electrical charge is not balanced. As defined, a complete cycle is less than 1 second.

2) Symmetric and asymmetric cycles (waveforms)

 a) *Symmetric* means that all of the waveform variables (amplitude, duration, and rate of rise and decay) are identical with respect to the isoelectric line for each half cycle (phase). Symmetric waveforms are always electrically balanced as they contain an equal but opposite charge in each half cycle (**Fig 5**).

 b) *Asymmetric* means that one or more of the waveform variables for each phase are unequal with respect to isoelectric line. Asymmetric waveforms may be electrically balanced or unbalanced (**Fig 5**).

3) Balanced vs unbalanced cycles (waveforms)

 a) *Balanced* means that the phase charges of each phase are equal. Balanced charges are commonly referred to as "zero net charge" (ZNC) or "zero net DC."

 b) *Unbalanced* means that the phase charges of the two phases in one cycle are unequal and the net charge is different from zero.

b. Time-dependent characteristics of AC

 1) For clinical purposes, *AC* is classified as the continuous flow of charges that must last at least one second and must cross over the isoelectric line at least twice within 1 second.

 2) *Frequency* describes the number of cycles per second and is usually expressed in hertz (Hz) or cycles per second.

 Note: We recognize the existence of several classifications for frequency (eg, physiologic, electrotherapeutic, and engineering). Frequency alone is not sufficient for determining the effects of AC. It is preferred that the specific frequency, rather than the relative classification, be stated. "Low," "medium," and "high" frequencies are examples of relative classifications and are not the preferred terms because the meaning and interpretation of these relative terms may differ among different biomedical disciplines.

 3) Rise and Decay Times

 a) *Rise time* is the time it takes the leading edge of the phase to increase from the baseline to peak amplitude of the phase (A in **Fig 5**).

 b) *Decay time* is the time it takes the trailing edge of the phase to return to the baseline from the peak amplitude of the phase (B in **Fig 5**).

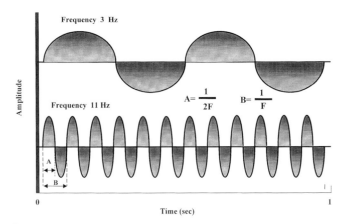

Figure 6
Alternating current (AC) inverse relationship between cycle duration (period) and the frequency (number of cycles per second) and their interdependence. The higher the frequency of AC, the shorter the duration of the cycle.

4) Period is the reciprocal of frequency and describes the time elapsed (duration) from a reference point of the cycle to the identical point of the next cycle. Therefore, a period equals one cycle's duration (B in **Fig 6**) and one half of the cycle equals one phase's duration (A in **Fig 6**). In therapeutic use, the cycle duration and the phase duration are expressed most commonly in microseconds (eg, 10 μs) or milliseconds (eg, 10 ms). In AC, there is an inverse relationship between frequency and period (cycle duration)—as frequency increases, cycle duration decreases. Conversely, as cycle duration increases, frequency decreases (**Fig 6**).

Note: As defined, AC has no intercycle or interphase intervals.

c. Amplitude-dependent characteristics of AC

1) *Amplitude* is the measure of the magnitude of current (or voltage) with reference to the isoelecteric line. Whenever possible, the current and voltage values should be specified.

Note: The term "intensity" frequently is used interchangeably with "amplitude" and "charge per pulse." To avoid confusion and inconsistency, the term "intensity" should never be used to describe current or voltage amplitude.

a) *Peak amplitude* is the highest amplitude of the current or voltage waveform. Amplitude is described as either "zero to peak" for one phase or "peak to peak" for one cycle (**Fig 7**).

b) *Root mean square (RMS) amplitude* represents the current (I_{RMS}) or voltage (V_{RMS}) applied over a specified length of time. The recommended time is 1 second. In AC, "peak current" and "I_{RMS} current" amplitudes are not the

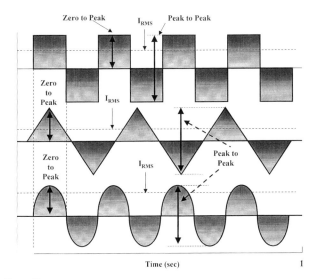

Figure 7
Amplitude-dependent characteristics of alternating current (AC). Upper graph, Rectangular symmetric AC. Middle graph, Triangular symmetric AC. Lower graph, Sinusoidal symmetric AC. Common amplitude specifications include "zero to peak" for each half-cycle, and "peak to peak" for each complete cycle or root mean square I$_{RMS}$. Depending on the shape, the I$_{RMS}$ may be higher or lower, but it is always less than the peak.

same. If delivered as a sine wave and depending on method of calculation, I$_{RMS}$ is either 65% or 70.7% of the peak amplitude and remains unchanged when the frequency is changed (**Fig 7**).

d. Time- and amplitude-dependent characteristics of AC

1) *Phase charge* (charge per phase) is the electrical charge within each half cycle of AC. It is calculated as the integrated sum of current amplitude multiplied by time (ie, area under the curve), and usually is measured in microcoulombs (**Fig 5**).

2) *Cycle charge* (charge per cycle) is the sum of the absolute value of the electrical charges of both phases of one cycle (period) of AC, also usually measured in microcoulombs.

e. Modulation of AC

Note: One or more of these modulations may occur simultaneously.

1) *Amplitude modulations* are variations in peak amplitude in a series of cycles. The modulations may be sequential or variable. A sequential increase and decrease of AC's amplitude within a few milliseconds is sometimes referred to as a "beat" (**Fig 8**).

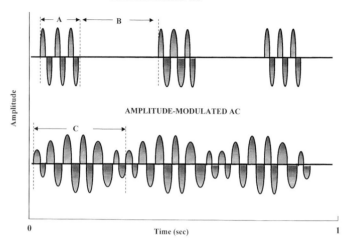

TIME-MODULATED AC

AMPLITUDE-MODULATED AC

Figure 8

Upper graph, Time-dependent modulation. Lower graph, Amplitude-dependent modulation of alternating current. A= burst duration, B= interburst interval, and C= beat duration. All three variables typically are measured in milliseconds. The number of bursts or beats delivered every second is termed "burst or "beat" frequency."

a) *Ramped AC* is the gradual increase (ramp up) or decrease (ramp down) of charge per phase over 1 second or longer (**Fig 11**). The AC phase charge can be increased by increasing peak current amplitude or decreasing fre-

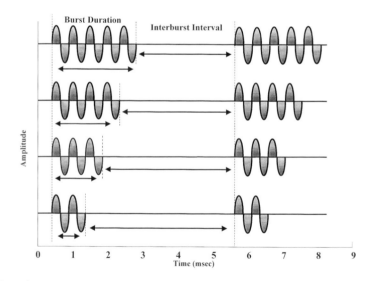

Figure 9

Time-dependent modulation of alternating current: variation in the number of cycles within a burst. Reduction of the number of cycles per burst shortens the burst duration and lengthens the interburst interval. Note that the number of bursts delivered per unit time remains unchanged.

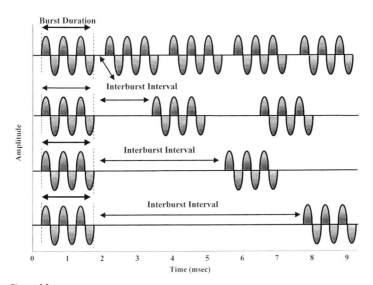

Burst Duration

Interburst Interval

Interburst Interval

Interburst Interval

Amplitude

0   1   2   3   4   5   6   7   8   9
Time (msec)

Figure 10

Time-dependent modulation of alternating current variation in the number of bursts per second (burst frequency) and the accompanied variation in the duration of the interburst intervals. Note that burst duration remains unchanged.

quency or both. The length of time from the ramp(s) onset to plateau and from plateau to termination, generally expressed in seconds, should be specified. Ramp modulation also has been called "rise time," but this is not the preferred term because *rise time* is a characteristic describing the rate of change in the amplitude of the leading edge of the individual phase of each cycle (**Fig 5**).

2) *Time modulations* are variations in the delivery pattern of a series of cycles.

   a) *Burst* is a group of two or more successive AC cycles, separated by a time interval without charge movement (interburst interval) and delivered at an identified frequency.

      i) *Burst duration* is the time elapsed from the beginning to the end of one burst. It is typically measured in milliseconds and is always less than 1 second (A in **Fig 8**).

      ii) *Interburst interval* is the time elapsed from the end of one burst to the beginning of the next burst. It is typically measured in milliseconds and is always less than 1 second (B in **Fig 8**). Interburst intervals can be increased by reducing the number of cycles contained in each burst (**Fig 9**) or by changing the number of bursts per second (**Fig 10**).

   b) *Interrupted AC* means that the AC ceases to flow for 1 second or longer. Once the AC is interrupted, the ON time and OFF times must be specified.

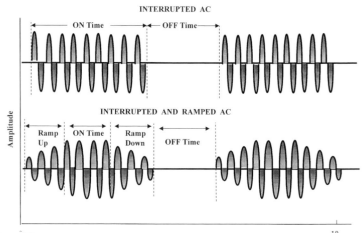

Figure 11

Time-dependent modulation of alternating current (AC). Upper graph, Interrupted AC. Lower graph, Amplitude- and time-modulated AC. Note that the time scale for ON, OFF and ramps is in seconds and that the ON time can be inclusive or exclusive of the ramp times. It is exclusive in this figure.

i) *ON time* is the time, typically measured in seconds, during which the AC (or bursts of AC) is delivered in a therapeutic application (**Fig 11**).

ii) *OFF time* is the time period that the AC is not flowing (typically measured in seconds) (**Fig 11**).

Note: The relationship between ON time and OFF time can be expressed as a ratio; for example, 10 seconds ON time and 20 seconds OFF time would produce a 1:2 ON time-to-OFF time ratio. ON time-to-OFF time ratios should not be used unless accompanied by an explicit description of the specific stimulation ON time and OFF time. Furthermore, the term "ON time" occasionally includes the ramp-up and ramp-down times and occasionally is exclusive of ramp times. To avoid confusion and inconsistency, the ramp-up and ramp-down times should be specified independently of the ON time. Likewise, the ON time should not include ramp-up or ramp-down times.

3. ***Pulsed Current or Pulsatile Current*** *(PC)* is the brief unidirectional or bidirectional flow of charged particles separated by a brief period of no flow. Pulsed current is commonly delivered as a series (train) of pulses. Each pulse is described by its waveform, rate of rise and decay, amplitude, duration, and frequency. Pulsed current also has been termed "pulsed AC," "interrupted AC," "pulsed DC," or "interrupted DC," but these are not preferred terms.

   a. Descriptive characteristics of PC

1) *Waveform* is the visual configuration of the current or voltage on the amplitude time plot. In PC, the waveform can be either monophasic (one phase) or biphasic (two opposing phases), each of which may be of different shapes (sine, square, triangular, spike, etc) (**Fig 12**).

2) *Phase* describes an electrical event that begins when the current (or voltage) departs from the isoelectric line and ends when it returns to the base line.

   a) *Monophasic* is a pulse that represents movement of charged particles in one direction for a very brief duration. The waveform of a monophasic pulse deviates in one direction from the isoelectric line and returns to the isoelectric line after a finite period of time. In a monophasic pulse, the amplitude and time-dependent characteristics of the phase and pulse are the same (**Fig 13**). By definition, the term "monophasic" is not applicable to a description of alternating currents.

   b) *Biphasic* is a pulse that represents bidirectional movement of charged particles for a very brief duration. The waveform of a biphasic pulse deviates in one direction from the isoelectric line and then deviates in the opposite direction from the isoelectric line. A biphasic waveform may be symmetric or asymmetric in reference to the isoelectric line. The characteristics of both phases should be fully described (**Fig 13**).

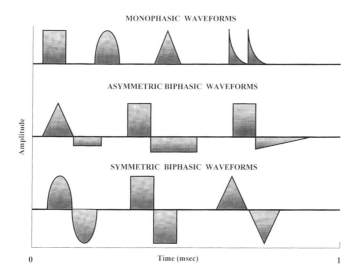

Figure 12

Examples of pulsed current (PC) waveforms. Upper graph, Different shapes of monophasic PC. Middle graph, Different shapes of asymmetric biphasic PC. Lower graph, Different shapes of symmetric biphasic PC. Biphasic symmetry is present when the amplitude and duration of both phases are identical. In asymmetrical biphasic, the charges of both phases may or may not be equal.

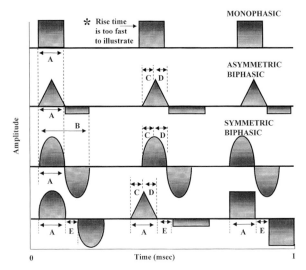

Figure 13

Time-dependent characteristics of pulsed current (PC). A=phase duration, B=pulse duration, C=rise time, D=fall time, and E=inter-phase (or intra-pulse) interval. Note that phase duration and pulse duration are synonymous in monophasic PC.

3) Symmetric and asymmetric waveforms

    a) *Symmetric* means that all of the waveform variables (amplitude, duration, and rate of rise and decay) are identical with respect to the isoelectric line for each phase. Symmetric waveforms are always electrically balanced (**Fig 13**).

    b) *Asymmetric* means that one or more of the waveform variables for each phase are unequal with respect to the isoelectric line. Asymmetric waveforms may be electrically balanced or unbalanced (**Fig 13**).

4) Balanced vs unbalanced waveforms

    a) *Balanced* means that the phase charges of each phase are equal. Balanced charges are commonly referred to as "zero net charge (ZNC)" or "zero net DC" (**Fig 14**).

    b) *Unbalanced* means that the phase charges of the two phases in one cycle are unequal and the net charge is different from zero (**Fig 14**).

b. Time-dependent characteristics of PC

1) Rise and decay times

    a) *Rise time* is the time it takes to go from the baseline to the peak amplitude of the phase (**C in Fig 13**).

---

b) *Decay time* is the time it takes to return to the baseline from the peak amplitude of the phase (**D in Fig 13**).

Note: If the shape is square, rise and fall times are extremely short (0.5 to 2 μs). For other shapes, such as sinusoidal, triangle, or exponential, the values typically are slightly longer.

2) *Phase duration* is the time elapsed between the beginning and the end of one phase of a pulse. In therapeutic use, phase duration is expressed most commonly in microseconds (eg, 10 μs) or milliseconds (eg, 10 ms) (**A in Fig 13**).

3) *Pulse duration* is the time elapsed between the beginning of the first phase and the end of second phase, and it may include the interphase interval within one pulse (**B in Fig 13**). In therapeutic use, pulse duration is expressed most commonly in microseconds (eg, 10 μs) or milliseconds (eg, 10 ms). Pulse duration cannot be used to describe AC waveforms.

Note: Pulse duration has been labeled "pulse width" on many stimulators. Since this parameter is time-dependent and not distance-dependent, the term "width" is incorrect.

4) *Interphase interval (intrapulse interval)* is the time elapsed between two successive

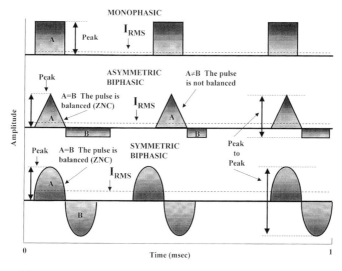

Figure 14
Amplitude- and time-dependent characteristics of pulsed current. Phase charge (A or B) is calculated as the peak current-time integral over the duration of each phase. Pulse charge is the absolute value summation of A+B. If A=B, the pulse charges are balanced and the pulse is said to have zero net charge (ZNC). If A≠B, the pulse is not balanced and the net charge is different than zero. Symmetric biphasic waveforms are always balanced and exhibit ZNC. Note that I_{RMS} can be calculated by adding the absolute values of all phase charges over 1 second (I_{RMS}=coulomb/s) and is always less than the peak current.

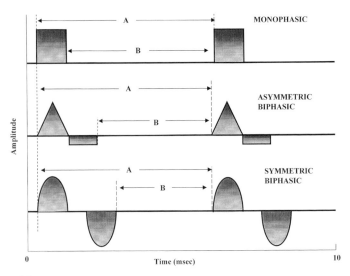

Figure 15
Additional time-dependent characteristics of pulsed current. A=period, and B=interpulse interval. Note that the time scale is in milliseconds.

phases of a biphasic pulse when no electrical activity occurs. The interphase interval must be shorter than the interpulse interval and is usually expressed in microseconds (**E in Fig 13**).

5) *Interpulse interval* is the time elapsed between two successive pulses and usually expressed in milliseconds (**B in Fig 15**).

6) *Frequency* describes the number of pulses per second (pps) for a pulsed current. The frequency of PC also has been commonly termed "pulse rate."

Note: Several classifications for frequency (eg, physiologic, electrotherapeutic, and engineering) are recognized in the literature. It is preferred that the specific frequency, rather than the relative classification, be stated. "Low," "medium," and "high" frequencies are examples of relative classifications. They are not the preferred terms because they do not disclose actual values and, therefore, are not informative.

7) *Period* is the reciprocal of frequency. The period is the time from a reference point of a pulse to the identical point of the next pulse (**A in Fig 15**). In pulsed currents, the period equals the pulse duration plus the interpulse interval.

c. Amplitude-dependent characteristics of PC

1) *Amplitude* is the measure of the magnitude of current (or voltage) with reference

to the isoelectric line. Whenever possible, the values for current and voltage should be specified.

Note: The term "intensity" frequently is used interchangeably with "amplitude" and "charge per pulse." To avoid confusion and inconsistency, the term "intensity" should not be used to describe current or voltage amplitude.

a) *Peak amplitude* is the highest amplitude of the current (or voltage) for a single phase. Amplitude is described as "zero to peak" for monophasic PC, or as either "zero to peak" or "peak to peak" for biphasic PC. "Peak-to-peak amplitude" is not a preferred way of expressing amplitude for an asymmetrical waveform because it does not give any information about the relative positive and negative amplitude (**Fig 14**).

b) *Root mean square (RMS) amplitude* represents the current (I_{RMS}) or voltage (V_{RMS}) applied over a specified length of time. The recommended time is 1 second. In PC, "peak current," and "I_{RMS} current" amplitudes are not the same and the latter typically is much lower because of the interpulse intervals (**Fig 14**). If used as defined, I_{RMS} will increase if any of the following will increase: peak current, phase duration, and pulse rate. I_{RMS} may be considered synonymous with the classic term "average current," but I_{RMS} is the preferred term. "Average current" can be appropriately applied to a monophasic but not to a biphasic waveform, whereas I_{RMS} can be applied to both.

d. Time- and amplitude-dependent characteristics of PC

1) *Phase charge* (charge per phase) is the charge within each phase (integrated sum of current amplitude multiplied by time; that is, area under the curve, measured in μQ) (**A in Fig 14**).

2) *Pulse charge* (charge per pulse) is the sum of the absolute value of the charges of both phases of the pulse as illustrated as A + B in **Fig 14**.

Note: In a monophasic waveform, the phase charge is equal to the pulse charge.

e. Modulations of PC

Note: One or more of these modulations may occur simultaneously.
1) *Amplitude modulations* are variations in the peak amplitude in a series of pulses. The modulation may be sequential or variable.

a) *Ramped PC* is the gradual increase (ramp up) or decrease (ramp down) of charge per phase over 1 second or longer. The PC phase charge can be increased by increasing peak current amplitude or by increasing phase duration, or both. A pulse-amplitude ramp sequence would be virtually indistinguishable from that of a phase-duration ramp. The time period from the ramp(s) onset to plateau and from plateau to termi-

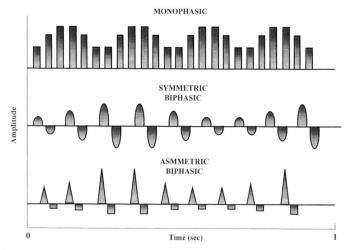

Figure 16

Amplitude-dependent modulation of pulsed current: repeated cyclic variations of pulse peak amplitude over a period of less than 1 second.

nation, generally expressed in seconds, should be specified (**Fig 16**). Ramp modulation also has been called "rise time." This is not the preferred terminology because rise time is a characteristic describing the rate of change in amplitude of the leading edge of the individual phase of each pulse (**C & D in Fig 13**).

b) *Reversing PC* is a term that applies only to a monophasic waveform. The reversal of polarity occurs typically after 1 second or longer. The time elapsed between reversal of polarity can vary from few microseconds to

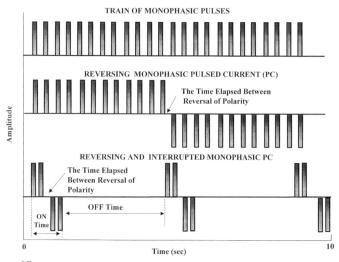

Figure 17

Polarity reversal of monophasic pulsed current. Upper graph, Unmodulated train of pulses. Middle graph, Polarity reversal. Lower graph, Polarity reversal plus interrupted modulation. Note that if the reversal occurs in less than 1 second, the time elapsed is termed "interpulse interval." If the time elapsed is longer than 1 second the term "interrupted PC" is recognized.

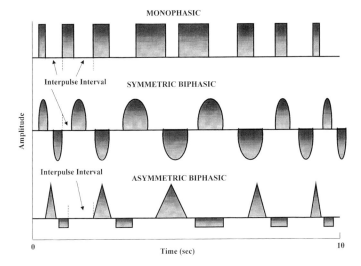

Figure 18

Time-dependent modulation of pulsed current: phase and pulse durations. Note that the pulse frequency (rate) is unaffected by the variation in duration. In contrast, the duration of the interpulse intervals is shortened as phase and pulse durations are prolonged.

several hundreds milliseconds and should be specified (**Fig 17**). If the time elapsed is longer than 1 second, the PC is considered interrupted and the OFF time must be specified (see "Interrupted PC" below).

2) *Timing modulations* are variations in the delivery pattern of a series of pulses.

   a) *Phase- or pulse-duration modulations* are variations in phase or pulse duration in a series of pulses. The modulation may be sequential or variable (**Fig 18**).

   b) *Burst* is two or more successive pulses separated by interburst intervals and delivered at an identified frequency (**Fig 19**).

      i) *Burst duration* is the time elapsed from the beginning to the end of one burst. Burst duration typically is measured in milliseconds and is always less than 1 second (**Fig 20**).

      ii) *Interburst interval* is the time elapsed from the end of one burst to the beginning of the next burst. Typically, it is measured in milliseconds and is always less than 1 second (**Fig 19**).

   c) *Interrupted PC* means the pulsed current ceases to flow for 1 second or longer. Once PC is interrupted, the ON time and OFF time must be specified.

      i) *ON time* is the time (typically measured in seconds) during which a train of pulses or bursts is delivered in a therapeutic application (**Fig 21**).

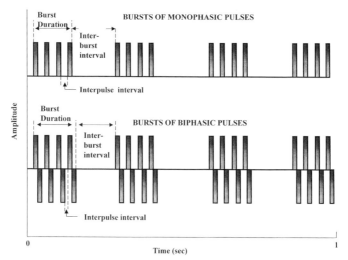

Figure 19

Time-dependent modulation of pulsed current: bursts of pulses. The duration of each burst is determined by the duration of the pulse's phases and the interpulse interval. The duration of the interburst interval is determined by the duration of each burst and the number of bursts per second.

    ii) *OFF time* is the time (typically measured in seconds) between trains of pulses or bursts (**Fig 21**).

    Note: The relationship between ON time and OFF time can be expressed as a ratio; for example, 10 seconds ON time and 20 seconds OFF time would

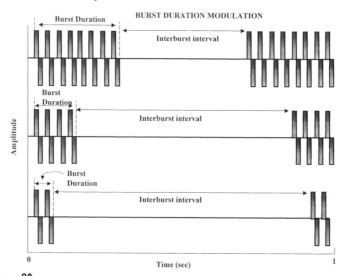

Figure 20

Time-dependent modulation of pulsed current: burst-duration modulation. The modulation is achieved by varying the number of pulses within each burst. Note that shortening the burst duration prolongs the interburst interval.

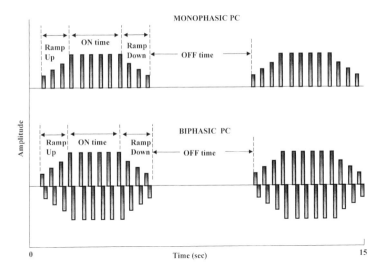

Figure 21

Time-dependent modulation of pulsed current: interrupted pulses. Note that the time scale for ON, OFF, and ramps is in seconds and that the ON time can be inclusive or exclusive of the ramp times. It is exclusive in this figure.

produce a 1:2 ON-time to OFF-time ratio. ON-time to OFF-time ratios should not be used unless accompanied by an explicit description of the specific stimulation ON time and OFF time. Furthermore, the term "ON time" occasionally includes the ramp-up and ramp-down times and occasionally is exclusive of ramp times. To avoid confusion and inconsistency, the ramp-up and ramp-down times should be specified independently of

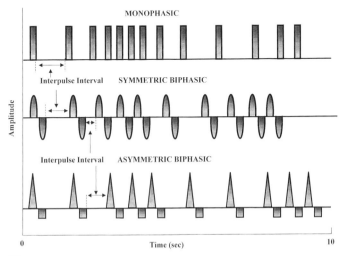

Figure 22

Pulse-frequency (-rate) modulation in pulsed current. Note that as frequency increases, the interpulse intervals are shortened.

Electrotherapeutic Terminology in Physical Therapy

the ON time. Likewise, the ON time should not include ramp-up or ramp-down times.

3) *Frequency modulations* are variations in frequency in a series of pulses. The modulations may be sequential or variable.

a) *Pulse-frequency (-rate) modulation* is the sequential or variable alteration of the number of pulses per second (pps). In PC, the change in pulse frequency occurs simultaneously with a change in the interpulse interval—the higher the pulse rate, the shorter the interpulse intervals (**Fig 22**).

b) *Burst-frequency modulation* is the sequential or variable alteration of the number of bursts per second (bps). In PC, the change in burst frequency occurs simultaneously with a change in the interburst interval—the higher the burst rate, the shorter the interburst intervals (**Fig 23**).

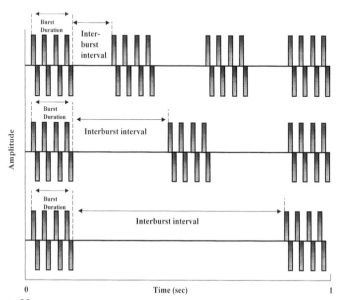

Figure 23

Burst-frequency modulation in pulsed current. Note that as burst frequency decreases, the interburst intervals are prolonged.

REFERENCES—Therapeutic Currents

Alon G, Kantor G, Ho HS. Effects of electrode size on basic excitatory responses and on selected stimulus parameters. *J Orthop Sports Phys Ther.* 1994;20(1):29-35.

Alon G, Kantor G, Ho HS. The effect of three types of surface electrodes on threshold excitation of human motor nerve. *J Clin Electrophysiol.* 1996;8:2-8.

Baker LL, Bowman BR, McNeal DR. Effects of waveform on comfort during neuromuscular electrical stimulation. *Clin Orthop.* 1988;(233):75-85.

Bowman BR, Baker LL. Effects of waveform parameters on comfort during transcutaneous neuromuscular electrical stimulation. *Ann Biomed Eng.* 1985;13(1):59-74.

Delitto A, Rose SJ. Comparative comfort of three waveforms used in electrically eliciting quadriceps femoris muscle contractions. *Phys Ther.* 1986;66(11):1704-1707.

Dumoulin C, et al. Pelvic-floor rehabilitation, I: comparison of two surface electrode placements during stimulation of the pelvic-floor musculature in women who are continent using bipolar interferential currents. *Phys Ther.* 1995;75(12):1067-1074.

Johnson MI, Ashton CH, Thompson JW. The consistency of pulse frequencies and pulse patterns of transcutaneous electrical nerve stimulation (TENS) used by chronic pain patients. *Pain.* 1991;44(3):231-234.

Kantor G, Alon G, Ho HS. The effects of selected stimulus waveforms on pulse and phase characteristics at sensory and motor thresholds. *Phys Ther.* 1994;74(10):951-962.

Kramer JF. Effect of electrical stimulation current frequencies on isometric knee extension torque. *Phys Ther.* 1987;67(1):31-38.

McCaffery M, Wolff M. Pain relief using cutaneous modalities, positioning, and movement. *Hosp J.* 1992;8(1-2):121-153.

Palmer ST, et al. Alteration of interferential current and transcutaneous electrical nerve stimulation frequency: effects on nerve excitation. *Arch Phys Med Rehabil.* 1999;80(9):1065-1071.

Szeto AY. Relationship between pulse rate and pulse width for a constant- intensity level of electrocutaneous stimulation. *Ann Biomed Eng.* 1985;13(5):373-383.

Ward AR, Robertson VJ. Variation in torque production with frequency using medium frequency alternating current. *Arch Phys Med Rehabil.* 1998;79(11):1399-1404.

III. Instrumentation Design and Application Considerations

A. Constant Current and Constant Voltage Stimulators

1. *Constant (or regulated) current instruments* provide current that flows at the same amplitude regardless of the impedance. By Ohm's law, the voltage varies proportionally to impedance to maintain the amplitude of current flow. (A specified impedance range exists over which the current is constant.)

2. *Constant (or regulated) voltage instruments* provide voltage in a predetermined manner that does not change in characteristics, regardless of the impedance or changes in impedance. By Ohm's law, the current flow varies inversely with impedance. (A specified impedance range exists over which the voltage is constant.)

Note: The design of a stimulator as a constant current or constant voltage affects the visual configuration of the waveform when applied to a human conductive medium (**Fig 24**). Therefore, reporting the stimulator design (constant voltage or constant current) and both voltage and current waveforms rather than just one is recommended.

B. Stimulation Electrodes

An electrode is an electrically conductive material used to transfer electrical charge to the tissue.

1. Types of electrodes

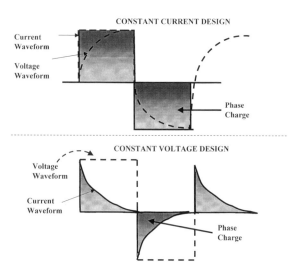

Figure 24
Constant-current and constant-voltage design of pulsed current. Due to the combined capacitive and resistive reactance of the biological conductive medium, the shapes and number of phases of the voltage and current waveforms are not the same.

a. *Surface (transcutaneous)* refers to electrodes that are placed in contact with the skin, usually through a coupling medium. Examples include metal (covered by wet cotton fabric, or sponge), carbonized silicon, and other conductive polymers.

b. *Invasive* refers to electrodes that penetrate the skin. Examples include percutaneous, epimyseal, and nerve-cuff electrodes.

2. A *coupling medium* is a substance used to enhance uniform conductivity at the electrode-skin interface. Examples include water, gel, and polymer.

3. Relationship between electrode surface area and current

a. With uniform electrode conductivity, the current density is inversely proportional to the electrode surface area. As the electrode contact area decreases, current density increases for a specified current.

b. Electrodes of larger surface area have lower impedance. The amount of electrode surface area is directly related to current flow. Thus, for a given voltage, the greater the surface area of the electrode, the greater the current flow. These relationships are a manifestation of Ohm's law.

Note: Absolute uniformity of electrode conductivity is an ideal situation that does not occur clinically. Therefore, electrodes that exhibit small variations from uniformity of conduction are acceptable.

4. Electrode configurations

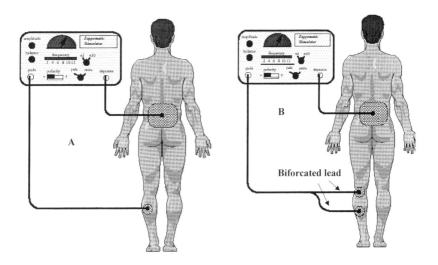

Figure 25
Monopolar technique of electrode placement. A=without biforcation, and B=with biforcation.

a. Description of electrode placement

The terms "monopolar," "bipolar," and "quadripolar" have been sources of confusion in electrotherapeutic applications; therefore, the preferred method of description is to describe the exact anatomical placement in relation to the target tissues and to state the exact size and dimensions of the electrode(s) used. A description of what has appeared in the literature in the past follows:

1) *Monopolar* means that one or more electrodes connected to one of the two circuit's leads are placed over the target tissue area where the greatest effect is desired and the other electrode(s) is connected to the second lead and placed at some distance from the target area (**Fig 25**). This other electrode has been labeled "dispersesive," "indifferent," "nontreatment," "reference," "return," or "inactive" in various publications. The source or rationale for choosing any of these labels in not known.

2) *Bipolar* means that all of the electrodes of one circuit are placed to affect the target area (**Fig 26**).

3) *Quadripolar or tetrapolar* means that four electrodes from two circuits are positioned so that the currents from these circuits will intersect within a target area between the electrodes (**Fig 27**).

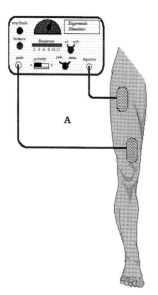
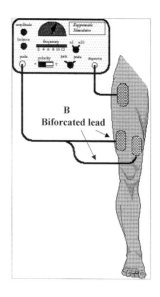

Figure 26
Bipolar technique of electrode placement. A=without biforcation, and B=with biforcation.

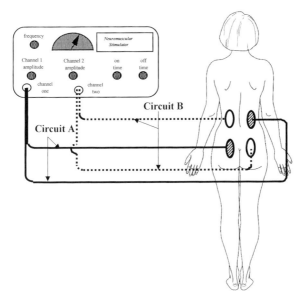

Figure 27

Quadripolar technique of electrode placement. This configuration typically is associated with Interferential Current (IC) and incorporates two circuits (see A and B) that are crossed in order to create the interference. IC is one way to generate amplitude modulation of alternating current.

b. *Ground (earth)* is an infinite electrical-charge source or accumulation. In AC-line-power-driven equipment, a reference is given to earth (ground) between the electrical stimulator and the power source. None of the electrodes in a patient circuit constitute a ground. Therefore, this term should not be used in association with patient electrode configurations in electrotherapy.

C. Description of Electrical Stimulation Applications

The purpose of the remainder of this publication is to clarify clinical and investigational application of electrical stimulation. The remaining material is included to acknowledge the existence of various terms used by practitioners, academicians, and manufacturers and to recommend the preferred terminology for categorizing or describing the clinical and investigational applications of therapeutic electrical stimulation.

Note: We acknowledge the existence of various ways of categorizing or describing the use of electrical stimulation, including those listed below. We suggest that uses of electrical stimulation be described in conjunction with treatment outcomes (goals). Examples may be the use of electrical stimulation for pain control, muscle strengthening, neuromuscular control, maintenance or improvement of joint mobility, resolution or reduction of acute or chronic edema, augmentation of peripheral circulation (arterial, venous, and lymphatic), and tissue repair. It is recognized that some clinical applications of electrical stimulation are not well substantiated by controlled studies; therefore, this section does not necessarily reflect evidence-based clinical efficacy for the applications that follow.

1. Clinical applications of electrotherapeutic currents

  a. Pain management
  Transcutaneous electrical nerve stimulation (TENS) is the use of externally applied electrical stimulation for pain management. The generic terms "TENS," "transcutaneous electrical stimulation (TES)," and "transcutaneous nerve stimulation (TNS)" all refer to electrical stimulation delivery systems that use surface electrodes. Based on clinical usage since the late 1960s, TENS customarily has been related to pain management. *Electroanalgesia* is a general term used to describe the outcome of using electrical stimulation to suppress pain.

  b. Neuromuscular dysfunction
  Muscle dysfunction typically includes weakness, decreased endurance (fatigue), and inability to contract at the correct magnitude, at the appropriate time, in concert with other muscles and with the external forces and moments (torque) applied to the system (motor control). Electrical stimulation has been applied, for the most part, to improve strength and motor control.

    1) Innervated muscle. *Neuromuscular electrical stimulation (NMES)* is the use of electrical stimulation for activation of muscles through stimulation of the intact peripheral motor nerves. The major treatment goals are to strengthen weak muscles and to help in the recovery of motor control. *Functional electrical stimulation (FES)* is the use of NMES to promote functional activities.

    2) Denervated muscle. *Electrical muscle stimulation (EMS)* is the use of electrical stimulation for direct activation of denervated muscle fibers in the absence of peripheral innervation. The major treatment goals are to retard muscle atrophy, and to improve local blood flow.

  c. Joint mobility
    1) NMES is used to induce repeated stretching of contracted, shortened soft tissues to regain, as a treatment goal, active and passive range of joint motion.

    2) TENS or NMES is used to mask the pain that may cause limited range of joint motion. The treatment goal is to regain normal joint range.

  d. Tissue repair
  Electrical stimulation for tissue repair (ESTR) involves the conduction of electrical current into the body to enhance microcirculation and protein synthe-

sis and to accelerate the healing process of slow-to-heal wounds. The primary goal of ESTR is to restore integrity of the connective and dermal tissues.

e. Acute and chronic edema (swelling)
Electrical current is used to affect blood vessel permeability, mobility of proteins, blood cells, and lymphatic flow through vasoconstriction or increased interstitial pressure. The treatment objectives are to curb edema formation and to accelerate the absorption rate in cases of both acute and chronic edema.

f. Peripheral blood flow
Electrical current is used to induce certain reflexes including but not limited to sensory-sympathetic or axon reflexes and to activate certain endogenous vasodilators such as vasoactive intestinal polypeptide (VIP) or calcitonin-gene-related peptide (CGRP). Electrical current also can be used to increase interstitial pressure to promote the clinical objective of augmenting arterial, venous, and lymphatic flow.

g. Urine and fecal incontinence
Electrical current is applied directly or indirectly to affect pelvic floor musculature by using penetrating or nonpenetrating surface electrodes. The clinical objectives include reducing pelvic pain, strengthening the pelvic floor musculature, and increasing sensation. Any or all of these impairments can be improved by electrical stimulation, and the treatment may lead to complete continence or considerable reduction of urge and stress incontinence.

h. Iontophoresis
Enhancement of transdermal delivery of pharmacological agents including but not limited to analgesic, anaesthetic, steroid and nonsteroid anti-inflammatory substances by electrical current. The most common clinical objectives are to reduce pain and edema associated with musculoskeletal disorders.

2. Vague terms
Some terms in common use do not describe electrotherapeutic instrumentation accurately and are not recommended for use in professional publications or presentations.

a. Trade or brand names should not be used to describe electrotherapeutic currents or specific treatment outcomes.

b. Individual characteristics of current should not be used in isolation as designations.

1) Waveform or current specifications

The most common misuse of terminology is related to waveform configurations.

Historically and technically, the term *galvanic* is used to describe an uninterrupted current that is synonymous with DC. The term *faradic* describes a specific type of pulsed current generated by rotation of a coiled wire in a magnetic field. The resultant waveform consists of an unbalanced, asymmetrical biphasic pulsed current (**Fig 13**). "Faradic" is not synonymous with "AC."

Therefore, the terms "galvanic" and "faradic" are not preferred terms for describing waveforms.

2) Relative amplitude specifications

High-voltage pulsed current (HVPC) and *high-volt pulsed galvanic stimulation (HVPGS)* both are inappropriate terms intended to refer to an electrical stimulator that typically has a monophasic waveform with a phase duration of usually less than 10 to 20 µs that employs a high-driving peak voltage (usually higher than 150 V). The term "HVPGS" is an inherent contradiction because galvanic current does not have pulses.

Low-voltage electrotherapeutic devices use longer pulse durations than HVPC and, consequently, require lower driving peak voltages (usually less than 150 V). All commercially available stimulators except HVPC devices fall into this category.

Low-intensity direct current (LIDC) is the term for therapeutic use of direct current of less than 1 mA. The preferred amplitude specification should reflect the voltage or current amplitude output range of the specific device.

Microcurrent is a general term used to describe a group of stimulators that deliver a pulsed current at a maximal peak amplitude of 999 micro amperes (less than 1 mA). These stimulators are designed to deliver low level of stimulation below the threshold of peripheral nerve excitation.

3) Frequency specifications

Frequency in general is described as the number of cycles per second (abbreviated Hz), or as the number of pulses per second (abbreviated pps).

In pain management with TENS, arbitrary classifications of "low" (less than 10 pps or Hz) and "high" (greater than 50 pps or Hz) frequency (rate) have been used.

In NMES, however, "low," "medium" (middle), and "high" frequency have assumed different meanings over the years. Low frequency usually is associated with the minimum frequency required to elicit titanic muscle contraction, but has included ranges of from 1 to 1,000 pps or Hz. Technically, medium frequency is defined as 1,000 to 10,000 pps or Hz; however, the extreme variability in physiological responses across these frequencies renders this classification impractical. This frequency range also has been erroneously called "high." Technically, *high frequency* is defined as greater than 100,000 pps or Hz and is used clinically for its thermal effects.

The preferred frequency specification should reflect the output (patient) circuit frequency ranges of the specific device, not the "carrier," or internal circuit, frequency.

4) Duty cycle specification

Duty cycle is the ratio of ON time to total time of trains of pulses or bursts. Duty cycle can be increased or decreased by changing burst duration (**Fig 21**) or interburst interval duration. (**Fig 22**) Duty cycle is expressed as a percentage using the relationships:

$$\text{Duty cycle} = \frac{\text{ON time}}{\text{ON time} + \text{OFF time}} \times 100$$

When describing duty cycle, the measured event (burst or train) should be specified. ON:OFF ratios (or the ratio of ON time to OFF time) have been erroneously equated with the term "duty-cycle."

Note: In isolation, the specification for waveforms, amplitude, frequency, or duty cycle is not sufficient to unambiguously characterize therapeutic stimulators.

c. Techniques

The following terms used to describe electrotherapeutic applications merely represent a "name-driven" treatment protocol or the current delivery through a specific electrode system. Because stimulation variables cannot be inferred or determined from these terms, the use of the following terms should be avoided.

• Russian technique, Russian stimulation
• Point stimulation (electroacupunture, hyperstimulation, electroacustimulation, acupoint stimulation, auriculotherapy, electrodiagnostic mapping)
• Acupuncture-like stimulation
• Conventional TENS
• Brief intense stimulation
• High frequency-low intensity
• Low frequency-high intensity
• Interferential Current (IC) therapy
• Microelectroneural stimulation (MENS)
• Lateral electrical stimulation for scoliosis (LESS)
• Therapeutic electrical stimulation (TES)

Appendix
Clinical-Outcome-Based Applications of Electrotherapeutic Currents

Research on electrotherapy spans hundreds of years and has been published in countless refereed journals. General suggestions or efficacy statements must be qualified first by scopes and limitations. This appendix provides a referenced outline of ranges of stimulus characteristics and parameters that have been used clinically to produce specific treatment outcomes. An attempt has been made to offer a list that is based solely on sampled data on clinical patients, rather than on animal or healthy subjects. The ranges indicated do not represent specific application guidelines. The parameters listed should not be incorporated arbitrarily in clinical applications of electrotherapy. Users of electrotherapy should refer to specific references in the professional scientific literature in order to safely and effectively employ electrotherapeutic interventions. (The reference list begins on page 44.)

Other scopes and limitations include the following:

1. Waveforms are not specified unless the electrical stimulation intervention requires the use of polarized current. In these cases the monophasic waveform is listed.

2. All applications involved use of either pulsed current (PC) or alternating current (AC), unless specified otherwise. Alternating current typically is used as amplitude- or time-modulated AC.

3. If ON and OFF times are not specified, the current is delivered as an uninterrupted train of pulses (PC) or bursts (AC).

4. Setting stimulation amplitude in the clinic can be better communicated among professionals if it is described in terms of patient or clinician perception or observation. Therefore, it is suggested that the terms "subsensory," "sensory," "motor," and "noxious" be used instead of "milliamps" and "volts."

As defined, *subsensory-level stimulation* occurs if the flow of current through a biological medium occurs at levels that are insufficient to generate action potentials in peripheral nerves. Subsensory level is achieved when the patient does not feel an electrically induced sensation.

Sensory-level stimulation is defined as the condition whereby the stimulus is sufficient to cause excitation of afferent nerve fibers whose action potentials propagate and reach the sensory cortex, leading to the subject's perception of tingling but without muscle contraction.

Motor-level stimulation occurs when the flow of charges is sufficient to depolarize efferent (motor) nerve fibers, or (in the absence of peripheral motor nerves) to depolarize denervated muscle fibers, leading to a detectable muscle contraction. The motor-level stimulation is always accompanied by sensory stimulation unless the patient suffers from sensory impairment or loss.

Noxious-level (painful-level) stimulation is defined as the physiological condition whereby the stimulus is sufficient to depolarize peripheral afferent nerve fibers whose propagated action potentials reach the sensory cortex and cause the perception of pain or discomfort, or both. Painful stimulation may be perceived concurrently with sensory-level or motor-level stimulation, or both. The patient typically describes the stimulus as painful or hurting.

The sensory, motor, and painful stimulation levels can each be described as minimal, moderate, or maximal perception.

The most common impairments to appear in the literature are the following:

Pain Management

1. Subsensory level stimulation
Committee members are aware of only one clinical research paper appearing in a refereed medical journal that provides some evidence to support the use of stimulation delivered below sensory perception to minimize perceived pain and joint stiffness in patient with osteoarthritis. (Zizic TM, et al. The treatment of osteoarthritis of the knee with pulsed electrical stimulation. *J Rheumatol.* 1995;22(9):1757-1761)

2. Sensory-level stimulation
Phase duration: 2 to 250 microseconds (μs)
Pulse duration: to 500 μs
Frequency: 0 to 200 pulses per second (pps) or cycles per second (Hz), or 50 to 200 bursts per second (bps)
Amplitude: sensory stimulation

3. Motor-level stimulation
Phase duration: 2 to 250 μs
Pulse duration: 4 to 500 μs
Burst duration: up to 10 milliseconds (ms)
Frequency: 1 to 5 pps (Hz) or 1 to 5 bps
Amplitude: motor stimulation resulting in twitch muscle contraction

4. Noxious- (painful-) level stimulation
Phase duration: up to 0.5 second (s)
Pulse duration: up to 1.0 s
Burst duration: up to 10 ms
Frequency: 1 to 200 pps (Hz) or 1 to 200 bps
Amplitude: painful stimulation to tolerance

Amelioration of Neuromuscular Dysfunction

1. Disuse atrophy
Phase duration: 1 to 300 µs
Note: Phase durations greater than 500 µs can be used but have been found to be less comfortable and require more phase/pulse charge for similar responses.
Pulse duration: 2 to 600 µs
Burst duration: up to 10 ms
Frequency: *fusion frequency*, which is defined as the frequency of motor-level stimulation at which a smooth tetanic muscle contraction is produced (generally ranging from 30 to 60 pps (Hz) for PC or from 30 to 60 bps for AC)
Amplitude: Motor stimulation resulting in muscle contraction (to maximal tolerance)
ON time: 5 to 15 s
OFF time: 5 to 60 s
Ramp up, down: 0.5 to 5 s

2. Motor control
Phase duration: 1 to 300 µs
Pulse duration: 2 to 600 µs
Burst duration: up to 10 ms
Frequency: 30 to 60 pps (Hz) for PC or 30 to 60 bps for AC (fusion frequency)
Amplitude: motor stimulation resulting in muscle contraction (to a level needed to Perform the task)
ON time: determined by the task
OFF time: determined by the task
Ramp up, down: determined by the task
Other desirable features: portable, battery operated, external trigger

Denervated Muscle

Electrical muscle stimulation (EMS)
Phase duration: greater than 1 ms (greater than denervated muscle chronaxie)
Pulse duration: greater than 2.0 ms
Frequency: 0.1 to 30 pps (Hz)
Amplitude: muscle contraction (to maximal tolerance)

Prevention or Resolution of Impaired Joint Mobility

Repeated stretching
Phase duration: 1 to 300 µs
Pulse duration: 2 to 600 µs
Burst duration: up to 10 ms
Frequency: 30 to 60 pps (Hz) for PC or from 30 to 60 bps for AC (fusion frequency)
Amplitude: motor stimulation resulting in muscle contraction sufficient to stretch the shortened soft tissues
ON time: 5 to 15 s

OFF time: 5 to 60 s
Ramp up, down: 1 to 5 s

Wound and Dermal Ulcer Healing
1. Stimulation into the wound
Waveform: monophasic
Phase duration: 2 to 50 μs
Pulse duration: 4 to 100 μs
Frequency: 100 to 125 pps (Hz)
Polarity: negative or positive over the wound
Amplitude: sensory stimulation

2. Stimulation away from the wound
Phase duration: 100 to 200 μs
Pulse duration: 200 to 400 μs
Burst duration: up to 10 ms
Frequency: 1 to 5 pps (Hz), or 1 to 5 bps
Amplitude: motor stimulation resulting in twitch contraction

Management of Acute and Chronic Edema (Swelling)
1. Acute edema
Waveform: monophasic
Phase duration: 2 to 50 μs
Pulse duration: 4 to 100 μs
Frequency: 100 to 125 pps (Hz)
Polarity: negative over swelling
Amplitude: sensory stimulation

2. Chronic edema
Phase duration: 50 to 300 μs
Pulse duration: 100 to 600 μs
Burst duration: up to 10 ms
Frequency: 30 to 60 pps (Hz) for PC or 30 to 60 bps for AC (fusion frequency)
Amplitude: motor stimulation resulting in muscle contraction (moderate)
ON time: 5 to 15 s
OFF time: 5 to 60 s
Ramp up, down: 0.5 to 5 s

Augmentation of Peripheral Blood Flow

1. Sensory-level stimulation
Phase duration: 2 to 250 µs
Pulse duration: 4 to 500 µs
Frequency: 4 to 100 pps (Hz)
Amplitude: sensory stimulation

2. Motor-level (twitch) stimulation
Phase duration: 100 to 200 µs
Pulse duration: 200 to 400 µs Burst duration: up to 10 ms
Frequency: 1 to 5 pps (Hz) or 1 to 5 bps
Amplitude: motor stimulation resulting in twitch contraction

3. Motor-level (tetanic) stimulation
Phase duration: 50 to 300 µs
Pulse duration: 100 to 600 µs
Burst duration: up to 10 ms
Frequency: 30 to 60 pps (Hz) for PC, or 30 to 60 bps for AC (fusion frequency)
Amplitude: motor stimulation resulting in muscle contraction (moderate)
ON time: 5 to 15 s
OFF time: 5 to 60 s
Ramp up, down: 0.5 to 5 s

Management of Incontinence

Phase duration: 20 to 300 µs
Pulse duration: 40 to 600 µs
Frequency: 5 to 50 pps (Hz)
Amplitude: motor stimulation resulting in muscle contraction (to maximal tolerance)
ON time: 5 s
OFF time: 10 s
Ramp up, down: 1 s

Iontophoresis (most studies used direct current)

A dose of up to 80 milliampere (mA)•min of direct current (DC) has been reported (eg, 4 mA applied for 20 min or 2 mA applied for 40 min will yield 80 mA•min)
Amplitude: less than or equal to 5 mA depending on electrode size and skin sensitivity
Polarity: either (+) or (-) depending on ionic component of the pharmacological agent

REFERENCES

The following selective reference list is restricted, with few exceptions, to clinical studies and to publications from the mid-1980s. The reader is encouraged to consult additional references by searching the Internet. One site to check is www.ncbi.nim.nih.gov/PubMed.

Pain Management

Abdel-Moty E, et al. Functional electrical stimulation in low back pain patients. *Pain Management.* 1988;1:258-263.

Bayindir O, et al. Use of transcutaneous electrical nerve stimulation in the control of postoperative chest pain after cardiac surgery. *J Cardiothorac Vasc Anesth.* 1991;5(6):589-591.

Benedetti F, et al. Control of postoperative pain by transcutaneous electrical nerve stimulation after thoracic operations [see comments in *Ann Thorac Surg.* 1997;63(3):608-610]. *Ann Thorac Surg.* 1997;63(3):773-776.

Borjesson M, et al. Transcutaneous electrical nerve stimulation in unstable angina pectoris. *Coron Artery Dis.* 1997;8(8-9):543-550.

Borjesson M. Visceral chest pain in unstable angina pectoris and effects of transcutaneous electrical nerve stimulation (TENS). A review. *Herz.* 1999;24(2):114-125.

Chabal C, et al. Long-term transcutaneous electrical nerve stimulation (TENS) use: impact on medication utilization and physical therapy costs. *Clin J Pain.* 1998;14(1):66-73.

Chantraine A, et al. Shoulder pain and dysfunction in hemiplegia: effects of functional electrical stimulation. *Arch Phys Med Rehabil.* 1999;80(3):328-331.

Chen L, et al. The effect of location of transcutaneous electrical nerve stimulation on postoperative opioid analgesic requirement: acupoint versus nonacupoint stimulation. *Anesth Analg.* 1998;87(5):1129-1134.

Chiu JH, et al. Effect of transcutaneous electrical nerve stimulation for pain relief on patients undergoing hemorrhoidectomy: prospective, randomized, controlled trial. *Dis Colon Rectum.* 1999;42(2):180-185.

Dawood MY, J. Ramos J. Transcutaneous electrical nerve stimulation (TENS) for the treatment of primary dysmenorrhea: a randomized crossover comparison with placebo TENS and ibuprofen. *Obstet Gynecol.* 1990;75(4):656-660.

Deyo RA, et al. A controlled trial of transcutaneous electrical nerve stimulation (TENS) and exercise for chronic low back pain [see comments in N Engl J Med. 1990;323(20):1423-1425]. *N Engl J Med.* 1990;322(23):1627-1634.

Donaldson D, Quarnstrom F, Jastak JT. The combined effect of nitrous oxide and oxygen and electrical stimulation during restorative dental treatment. *J Am Dent Assoc.* 1989;118(6):733-736.

Fishbain DA, et al. Transcutaneous electrical nerve stimulation (TENS) treatment outcome in long-term users. *Clin J Pain.* 1996;12(3):201-214.

Fisher WW, et al. Reductions in self-injury produced by transcutaneous electrical nerve stimulation. *J Appl Behav Anal.* 1998;31(3):493-496.

Forster EL, et al. Effect of TENS on pain, medications, and pulmonary function following coronary artery bypass graft surgery. *Chest.* 1994;106(5):1343-1348.

Gadsby JG, Flowerdew MW. Transcutaneous electrical nerve stimulation and acupuncture-like transcutaneous electrical nerve stimulation for chronic low back pain. *Cochrane Database Syst Rev.* 2000;2:CD000210.

Gemignani G, et al. Transcutaneous electrical nerve stimulation in ankylosing spondylitis: a double-blind study. *Arthritis Rheum.* 1991;34(6):788-789. Letter.

Graff-Radford SB, et al. Effects of transcutaneous electrical nerve stimulation on myofascial pain and trigger point sensitivity. *Pain.*1989;37(1):1-5.

Grant DJ, et al. A randomized comparative trial of acupuncture versus transcutaneous electrical nerve stimulation for chronic back pain in the elderly. *Pain.* 1999;82(1):9-13.

Grechko VE, Borisova EG. Use of transcutaneous electrical nerve stimulation in the complex treatment of glossalgia. *Neurosci Behav Physiol.* 1996;26(6):584-586.

Guelrud M, et al. Transcutaneous electrical nerve stimulation decreases lower esophageal sphincter pressure in patients with achalasia. *Dig Dis Sci.* 1991;36(8):1029-1033.

Guieu R, et al. Pain relief achieved by transcutaneous electrical nerve stimulation and/or vibratory stimulation in a case of painful legs and moving toes. *Pain.* 1990;42(1):43-48.

Guieu R, Tardy-Gervet MF, Roll JP. Analgesic effects of vibration and transcutaneous electrical nerve stimulation applied separately and simultaneously to patients with chronic pain. *Can J Neurol Sci.* 1991;18(2):113-119.

Hamza MA, et al. Effect of the frequency of transcutaneous electrical nerve stimulation on the postoperative opioid analgesic requirement and recovery profile. *Anesthesiology.* 1999;91(5):1232-1238.

Hargreaves A, Lander J. Use of transcutaneous electrical nerve stimulation for postoperative pain. *Nurs Res.* 1989;38(3):159-161.

Harvey M, Elliott M. Transcutaneous electrical nerve stimulation (TENS) for pain management during cavity preparations in pediatric patients. *ASDC J Dent Child.* 1995;62(1):49-51.

Herman E, et al. A randomized controlled trial of transcutaneous electrical nerve stimulation (CODE-TRON) to determine its benefits in a rehabilitation program for acute occupational low back pain. *Spine.* 1994;19(5):561-568.

Jayme MK, et al. Effectivity of the electronic dental anesthesia in controlling pain caused by local anesthetic injections. *J Philipp Dent Assoc.* 1998;50(3):39-52.

Jensen H, Zesler R, Christensen T. Transcutaneous electrical nerve stimulation (TNS) for painful osteoarthrosis of the knee. *Int J Rehabil Res.* 1991;14(4):356-358.

Johnson MI, Ashton CH, Thompson JW. An in-depth study of long-term users of transcutaneous electrical nerve stimulation (TENS): implications for clinical use of TENS. *Pain.* 1991;44(3):221-229.

Kaplan B, et al. Transcutaneous electrical nerve stimulation (TENS) for adjuvant pain-relief during labor and delivery. *Int J Gynaecol Obstet.* 1998; 60(3):251-255.

Kruger LR, van der Linden WJ, Cleaton-Jones PE. Transcutaneous electrical nerve stimulation in the treatment of myofascial pain dysfunction. *S Afr J Surg.* 1998;36(1):35-38.

Lampl C, Kreczi T, Klingler D. Transcutaneous electrical nerve stimulation in the treatment of chronic pain: predictive factors and evaluation of the method. *Clin J Pain.* 1998;14(2):134-142.

Leandri M, et al. Comparison of TENS treatments in hemiplegic shoulder pain. *Scand J Rehabil Med.* 1990;22(2):69-71.

Lee EW, et al. The role of transcutaneous electrical nerve stimulation in management of labour in obstetric patients. *Asia Oceania J Obstet Gynaecol.* 1990;16(3):247-254.

Leijon G, Boivie J. Central post-stroke pain—the effect of high and low frequency TENS. *Pain.* 1989;38(2):187-191.

Lewers D, et al. Transcutaneous electrical nerve stimulation in the relief of primary dysmenorrhea. *Phys Ther.* 1989;69(1):3-9.

Lewis SM, et al. Effects of auricular acupuncture-like transcutaneous electric nerve stimulation on pain levels following wound care in patients with burns: a pilot study. *J Burn Care Rehabil.* 1990;11(4):322-329.

Magarian GJ, Leikam B, Palac R. Transcutaneous electrical nerve stimulation (TENS) for treatment of severe angina pectoris refractory to maximal medical and surgical management-a case report. *Angiology.* 1990;41(5):408-411.

Mannheimer C, Emanuelsson H, and Waagstein F. The effect of transcutaneous electrical nerve stimulation (TENS) on catecholamine metabolism during pacing-induced angina pectoris and the influence of naloxone. *Pain.* 1990;41(1):27-34.

McDowell BC, et al. Comparative analgesic effects of H-wave therapy and transcutaneous electrical nerve stimulation on pain threshold in humans. *Arch Phys Med Rehabil.* 1999;80(9):1001-1004.

Meyler WJ, de Jongste MJ, Rolf CA. Clinical evaluation of pain treatment with electrostimulation: a study on TENS in patients with different pain syndromes. *Clin J Pain.* 1994;10(1):22-27.

Milsom I, Hedner N, Mannheimer C. A comparative study of the effect of high-intensity transcutaneous nerve stimulation and oral naproxen on intrauterine pressure and menstrual pain in patients with primary dysmenorrhea. *Am J Obstet Gynecol.* 1994;170(1 pt 1):123-129.

Moore SR, Shurman J. Combined neuromuscular electrical stimulation and transcutaneous electrical nerve stimulation for treatment of chronic back pain: a double-blind, repeated measures comparison. *Arch Phys Med Rehabil.* 1997;78(1):55-60.

Peeker R, Fall M. Treatment guidelines for classic and non-ulcer interstitial cystitis. *Int Urogynecol J Pelvic Floor Dysfunct.* 2000;11(1):23-32.

Quarnstrom FC, Milgrom P. Clinical experience with TENS and TENS combined with nitrous oxide-oxygen: report of 371 patients. *Anesth Prog.* 1989;36(2):66-69.

Reichelt O, et al. Effective analgesia for extracorporeal shock wave lithotripsy: transcutaneous electrical nerve stimulation. *Urology.* 1999;54(3):433-436.

Robaina FJ, et al. Transcutaneous electrical nerve stimulation and spinal cord stimulation for pain relief in reflex sympathetic dystrophy. *Stereotact Funct Neurosurg.* 1989;52(1):53-62.

Sanderson JE. Electrical neurostimulators for pain relief in angina [see comments in *Br Heart J.* 1991;65(4):234-235]. *Br Heart J.* 1990;63(3):141-143.

Somers DL, Somers MF. Treatment of neuropathic pain in a patient with diabetic neuropathy using transcutaneous electrical nerve stimulation applied to the skin of the lumbar region. *Phys Ther.* 1999;79(8):767-775.

teDuits E, et al. The effectiveness of electronic dental anesthesia in children. *Pediatr Dent.* 1993;15(3):191-6.

Torres WE, et al. The use of transcutaneous electrical nerve stimulation during the biliary lithotripsy procedure. *J Stone Dis.* 1992;4(1):41-45.

Tsen LC, et al. Transcutaneous electrical nerve stimulation does not augment combined spinal epidural labour analgesia. *Can J Anaesth.* 2000;47(1):38-42.

Tulgar M, et al. Comparative effectiveness of different stimulation modes in relieving pain, II: a double-blind controlled long-term clinical trial. *Pain.* 1991;47(2):157-162.

van der Ploeg JM, et al. Transcutaneous nerve stimulation (TENS) during the first stage of labour: a randomized clinical trial. *Pain.* 1996;68(1):75-78.

Walsh IK, Johnston RS, Keane PF. Transcutaneous sacral neurostimulation for irritative voiding dysfunction. *Eur Urol.* 1999;35(3):192-196.

Wang B, et al. Effect of the intensity of transcutaneous acupoint electrical stimulation on the postoperative analgesic requirement. *Anesth Analg.* 1997;85(2):406-413.

Wang WC, George SL, Wilimas JA. Transcutaneous electrical nerve stimulation treatment of sickle cell pain crises. *Acta Haematol.* 1988;80(2):99-102.

Werner S, et al. Electrical stimulation of vastus medialis and stretching of lateral thigh muscles in patients with patello-femoral symptoms. *Knee Surg Sports Traumatol Arthrosc.* 1993;1(2):85-92.

Wilder RT, et al. Reflex sympathetic dystrophy in children. Clinical characteristics and follow-up of seventy patients. *J Bone Joint Surg Am.* 1992;74(6):910-919.

Orthopedics Neuromuscular Impairments

Abdel-Moty E, et al. Functional electrical stimulation in low back pain patients. *Pain Management.* 1988;1:258-263.

Abdel-Moty E, et al. Functional electrical stimulation treatment of postradiculopathy associated muscle weakness. *Arch Phys Med Rehabil.* 1994;75:680-686.

Anderson AF, Lipscomb AB. Analysis of rehabilitation techniques after anterior cruciate reconstruction. *Am J Sports Med.* 1989;17(2):154-160.

Arvidsson I, et al. Prevention of quadriceps wasting after immobilization: an evaluation of the effect of electrical stimulation. *Orthopedics.* 1986;9(11):1519-1528.

Currier DP, et al. Effects of electrical and electromagnetic stimulation after anterior cruciate ligament reconstruction. *J Orthop Sports Phys Ther.* 1993;17(4):177-184.

Delitto A, et al. Electrical stimulation versus voluntary exercise in strengthening thigh musculature after anterior cruciate ligament surgery [see erratum in *Phys Ther.* 1988;68(7):1145]. *Phys Ther.* 1988;68(5):660-663.

Draper V, Ballard L. Electrical stimulation versus electromyographic biofeedback in the recovery of quadriceps femoris muscle function following anterior cruciate ligament surgery [see comments in *Phys Ther.* 1991;71(10):762]. *Phys Ther.* 1991;71(6):455-461; discussion 461-464.

Eriksson E, Haggmark T. Comparison of isometric muscle training and electrical stimulation supplementing isometric muscle training in the recovery after major knee ligament surgery: a preliminary report. *Am J Sports Med.* 1979;7(3):169-171.

Gibson JN, Smith K, Rennie MJ. Prevention of disuse muscle atrophy by means of electrical stimulation: maintenance of protein synthesis. *Lancet.* 1988;2(8614):767-770.

Gould N, et al. Transcutaneous muscle stimulation to retard disuse atrophy after open meniscectomy. *Clin Orthop.* 1983;(178):190-197.

Kidd GL, Electrical stimulation for disuse muscle atrophy. *Lancet.* 1988;2(8618):1025. Letter.

Lieber RL, Silva PD, Daniel DM. Equal effectiveness of electrical and volitional strength training for quadriceps femoris muscles after anterior cruciate ligament surgery. *J Orthop Res.* 1996;14(1):131-138.

Martin TP, et al. The influence of functional electrical stimulation on the properties of vastus lateralis fibres following total knee arthroplasty. *Scand J Rehabil Med.* 1991;23(4):207-210.

Matheson GO, et al. Force output and energy metabolism during neuromuscular electrical stimulation: a 31P-NMR study. *Scand J Rehabil Med.* 1997;29(3):175-180.

Morrissey MC, et al. The effects of electrical stimulation on the quadriceps during postoperative knee immobilization. *Am J Sports Med.* 1985;13(1):40-45.

Oldham JA, Stanley JK. Rehabilitation of atrophied muscle in the rheumatoid arthritic hand: a comparison of two methods of electrical stimulation. *J Hand Surg Br.* 1989;14(3):294-297.

Paternostro-Sluga T, et al. Neuromuscular electrical stimulation after anterior cruciate ligament surgery. *Clin Orthop.* 1999;(368):166-175.

Petterson T, et al. The use of patterned neuromuscular stimulation to improve hand function following surgery for ulnar neuropathy. *J Hand Surg Br.* 1994;19(4):430-433.

Quittan M, et al. Strength improvement of knee extensor muscles in patients with chronic heart failure by neuromuscular electrical stimulation. *Artif Organs.* 1999;23(5):432-435.

Rizk TE, Park SJ. Transcutaneous electrical nerve stimulation and extensor splint in linear scleroderma knee contracture. *Arch Phys Med Rehabil.* 1981;62(2):86-8.

Sisk TD, et al. Effect of electrical stimulation on quadriceps strength after reconstructive surgery of the anterior cruciate ligament. *Am J Sports Med.* 1987;15(3):215-220.

Snyder-Mackler L, Binder-Macleod SA, Williams PR. Fatigability of human quadriceps femoris muscle following anterior cruciate ligament reconstruction. *Med Sci Sports Exerc.* 1993;25(7):783-789.

Snyder-Mackler L, et al. Electrical stimulation of the thigh muscles after reconstruction of the anterior cruciate ligament. Effects of electrically elicited contraction of the quadriceps femoris and hamstring muscles on gait and on strength of the thigh muscles. *J Bone Joint Surg Am.* 1991;73(7):1025-1036.

Snyder-Mackler L, et al. Strength of the quadriceps femoris muscle and functional recovery after reconstruction of the anterior cruciate ligament. A prospective, randomized clinical trial of electrical stimulation. *J Bone Joint Surg Am.* 1995;77(8):1166-1173.

Snyder-Mackler L, et al. Use of electrical stimulation to enhance recovery of quadriceps femoris muscle force production in patients following anterior cruciate ligament reconstruction [see comments in *Phys Ther.* 1995;75(3):237-238]. *Phys Ther.* 1994;74(10):901-907.

Wigerstad-Lossing I, et al. Effects of electrical muscle stimulation combined with voluntary contractions after knee ligament surgery. *Med Sci Sports Exerc.* 1988;20(1):93-98.

You JM, Landymore RW, Fris J. Delayed stimulation of the latissimus dorsi may result in disuse atrophy. *Ann Thorac Surg.* 1997;64(2):404-408; discussion 408-409.

Central Nervous System (CNS)

Alon G, et al. Efficacy of a hybrid upper limb neuromuscular electrical stimulation system in lessening selected impairments and dysfunctions consequent to cerebral damage. *J Neurol Rehabil.* 1998;12:73-80.

Baker LL, Parker K. Neuromuscular electrical stimulation of the muscles surrounding the shoulder. *Phys Ther.* 1986;66(12):1930-1937.

Bogataj U, et al. Enhanced rehabilitation of gait after stroke: a case report of a therapeutic approach using multichannel functional electrical stimulation. *IEEE Trans Rehabil Eng.* 1997;5(2):221-232.

Bogataj U, et al. Restoration of gait during two to three weeks of therapy with multichannel electrical stimulation. *Phys Ther.* 1989;69(5):319-327.

Burridge JH, et al. The effects of common peroneal stimulation on the effort and speed of walking: a randomized controlled trial with chronic hemiplegic patients. *Clin Rehabil.* 1997;11(3):201-210.

Canavero S, et al. Painful supernumerary phantom arm following motor cortex stimulation for central poststroke pain: case report. *J Neurosurg.* 1999;91(1):121-123.

Cauraugh J, et al. Chronic motor dysfunction after stroke: recovering wrist and finger extension by electromyography-triggered neuromuscular stimulation. *Stroke.* 2000;31(6):1360-1364.

Chae J, Hart R. Comparison of discomfort associated with surface and percutaneous intramuscular electrical stimulation for persons with chronic hemiplegia. *Am J Phys Med Rehabil.* 1998;77(6):516-522.

Chantraine A, et al. Shoulder pain and dysfunction in hemiplegia: effects of functional electrical stimulation. *Arch Phys Med Rehabil.* 1999;80(3):328-331.

Cozean CD, Pease WS, Hubbell SL. Biofeedback and functional electric stimulation in stroke rehabilitation. *Arch Phys Med Rehabil.* 1988;69(6):401-405.

Daly JJ, et al. Therapeutic neural effects of electrical stimulation. *IEEE Trans Rehabil Eng.* 1996;4(4): 218-230.

Daly JJ, Ruff RL. Electrically induced recovery of gait components for older patients with chronic stroke. *Am J Phys Med Rehabil.* 2000;79(4):349-360.

Dewald JP, Given JD, Rymer WZ. Long-lasting reductions of spasticity induced by skin electrical stimulation. *IEEE Trans Rehabil Eng.* 1996;4(4):231-242.

Dimitrijevic MM, Soroker N. Mesh-glove, II: modulation of residual upper limb motor control after stroke with whole-hand electric stimulation. *Scand J Rehabil Med.* 1994;26(4):187-190.

Dimitrijevic, M.M., Mesh-glove, I: a method for whole-hand electrical stimulation in upper motor neuron dysfunction. *Scand J Rehabil Med.* 1994;26(4):183-186.

Faghri PD, et al. Electrical stimulation-induced contraction to reduce blood stasis during arthroplasty. *IEEE Trans Rehabil Eng.* 1997;5(1):62-69.

Faghri PD, et al. The effects of functional electrical stimulation on shoulder subluxation, arm function recovery, and shoulder pain in hemiplegic stroke patients. *Arch Phys Med Rehabil.* 1994;75(1):73-79.

Feketa VP. Application of biomechanical stimulation of lower extremity muscles in the treatment of patients with hypertension [in Russian]. *Kardiologiia.* 1992;32(11-12):23-25.

Francisco G, et al. Electromyogram-triggered neuromuscular stimulation for improving the arm function of acute stroke survivors: a randomized pilot study. *Arch Phys Med Rehabil.* 1998;79(5):570-575.

Glanz M, et al. Functional electrostimulation in poststroke rehabilitation: a meta- analysis of the randomized controlled trials. *Arch Phys Med Rehabil.* 1996;77(6):549-553.

Granat MH, et al. Peroneal stimulator: evaluation for the correction of spastic drop foot in hemiplegia. Arch Phys Med Rehabil. 1996;77(1):19-24.

Herregodts P, et al. Cortical stimulation for central neuropathic pain: 3-D surface MRI for easy determination of the motor cortex. *Acta Neurochir Suppl.* 1995;64:132-135.

Hesse S, et al. Botulinum toxin type A and short-term electrical stimulation in the treatment of upper limb flexor spasticity after stroke: a randomized, double-blind, placebo-controlled trial. *Clin Rehabil.* 1998;12(5):381-388.

Hooker SP, et al. Physiologic responses to prolonged electrically stimulated leg-cycle exercise in the spinal cord injured. *Arch Phys Med Rehabil.* 1990;71(11):863-869.

Hummelsheim H, Maier-Loth ML, Eickhof C. The functional value of electrical muscle stimulation for the rehabilitation of the hand in stroke patients. *Scand J Rehabil Med.* 1997;29(1):3-10.

Kameyama J, et al. Restoration of shoulder movement in quadriplegic and hemiplegic patients by functional electrical stimulation using percutaneous multiple electrodes. *Tohoku J Exp Med.* 1999;187(4):329-337.

Kraft GH, Fitts SS, Hammond MC. Techniques to improve function of the arm and hand in chronic hemiplegia. *Arch Phys Med Rehabil.* 1992;73(3):220-227.

Kralj A, Acimovic R, Stanic U. Enhancement of hemiplegic patient rehabilitation by means of functional electrical stimulation. *Prosthet Orthot Int.* 1993;17(2):107-114.

Leijon G, Boivie J. Central post-stroke pain—the effect of high and low frequency TENS. *Pain.* 1989;38(2):187-191.

Linn SL, Granat MH, Lees KR. Prevention of shoulder subluxation after stroke with electrical stimulation. *Stroke.* 1999;30(5):963-968.

Macheret EL, D'Iachenko O, Korkushko OO. The treatment of patients with chronic cerebral circulatory failure by using laser puncture and the microclimate of the biotron [in Ukrainian]. *Lik Sprava.* 1996(7-9):142-145.

Macheret EL, Samosiuk IZ, Shuman Iu A. Activation of motor function in patients with cerebral paresis and paralysis after electric stimulation [in Russian]. *Vrach Delo.* 1988(4):76-77

Magnusson M, Johansson K, Johansson BB. Sensory stimulation promotes normalization of postural control after stroke. *Stroke.* 1994;25(6):1176-1180.

Magovern GJ, et al. Paced skeletal muscle for dynamic cardiomyoplasty. *Ann Thorac Surg.* 1988;45(6):614-619.

Malezic M, et al. Application of a programmable dual-channel adaptive electrical stimulation system for the control and analysis of gait. *J Rehabil Res Dev.* 1992;29(4):41-53.

Oh JH, Badhwar V, Chiu RC, Hemodynamic response to in situ latissimus dorsi muscle stimulation: implications in dynamic cardiomyoplasty. *J Card Surg.* 1997;12(5):354-359.

Pambianco G, Orchard T, Landau P. Deep vein thrombosis: prevention in stroke patients during rehabilitation. *Arch Phys Med Rehabil.* 1995;76(4):324-330.

Pandyan AD, Granat MH, Stott DJ. Effects of electrical stimulation on flexion contractures in the hemiplegic wrist. *Clin Rehabil.* 1997;11(2):123-130.

Peyron R, et al. Electrical stimulation of precentral cortical area in the treatment of central pain: electrophysiological and PET study. *Pain.* 1995;62(3):275-286.

Popovic D, et al. Optimal control of walking with functional electrical stimulation: a computer simulation study. *IEEE Trans Rehabil Eng.* 1999;7(1):69-79.

Potisk KP, Gregoric M, Vodovnik L. Effects of transcutaneous electrical nerve stimulation (TENS) on spasticity in patients with hemiplegia. *Scand J Rehabil Med.* 1995;27(3):169-174.

Powell J, et al. Electrical stimulation of wrist extensors in poststroke hemiplegia. *Stroke.* 1999;30(7):1384-1389.

Prada GT, R, Treatment of the neglect syndrome in stroke patients using a contingency electrical stimulation. *Clin Rehabil.* 1995;9:304-313.

Prochazka A, et al. The bionic glove: an electrical stimulator garment that provides controlled grasp and hand opening in quadriplegia. *Arch Phys Med Rehabil.* 1997;78(6):608-614.

Quittan M, et al. Strength improvement of knee extensor muscles in patients with chronic heart failure by neuromuscular electrical stimulation. *Artif Organs.* 1999;23(5):432-435.

Raymond J, et al. Cardiovascular responses to an orthostatic challenge and electrical-stimulation-induced leg muscle contractions in individuals with paraplegia. *Eur J Appl Physiol.* 1999;80(3):205-212.

Richards L, Pohl P. Therapeutic interventions to improve upper extremity recovery and function. *Clin Geriatr Med.* 1999;15(4):819-832.

Rorsman I, Magnusson M, Johansson BB. Reduction of visuo-spatial neglect with vestibular galvanic stimulation. *Scand J Rehabil Med.* 1999;31(2):117-124.

Siebner HR, et al. Changes in handwriting resulting from bilateral high-frequency stimulation of the subthalamic nucleus in Parkinson's disease. *Mov Disord.* 1999;14(6):964-971.

Slepushkina TG, Minenkov AA, Strel'tsova EN. The use of interference currents with patients in the late recovery period after an ischemic stroke and with patients with cervical osteochondrosis and a pain syndrome [in Russian]. *Vopr Kurortol Fizioter Lech Fiz Kult.* 1995;(2):16-18.

Smith LE. Restoration of volitional limb movement of hemiplegics following patterned functional electrical stimulation. *Percept Mot Skills.* 1990;71(3 pt 1):851-861.

Sonde L, et al. Low TENS treatment on post-stroke paretic arm: a three-year follow-up. *Clin Rehabil.* 2000;14(1):14-19.

Sonde L, et al. Stimulation with low frequency (1.7 Hz) transcutaneous electric nerve stimulation (lowtens) increases motor function of the post-stroke paretic arm. *Scand J Rehabil Med.* 1998;30(2):95-99.

Stein RB, et al. Estimating mechanical parameters of leg segments in individuals with and without physical disabilities. *IEEE Trans Rehabil Eng.* 1996;4(3):201-211.

Sumin AN, et al. Pilot experience with skeletal muscles electrostimulation in rehabilitation of patients with complicated myocardial infarction [in Russian]. *Ter Arkh.* 1999;71(12):18-20.

Tasker RR, Vilela Filho O. Deep brain stimulation for neuropathic pain. *Stereotact Funct Neurosurg.* 1995;65(1-4):122-124.

Taylor P, et al. Clinical audit of 5 years provision of the Odstock dropped foot stimulator. *Artif Organs.* 1999;23(5):440-442.

Taylor PN, et al. Clinical use of the Odstock dropped foot stimulator: its effect on the speed and effort of walking. *Arch Phys Med Rehabil.* 1999;80(12):1577-1583.

Taylor PN, et al. Patients' perceptions of the Odstock dropped foot stimulator (ODFS). *Clin Rehabil.* 1999;13(5):439-446.

Tekeoglu Y, Adak B, Goksoy T. Effect of transcutaneous electrical nerve stimulation (TENS) on Barthel Activities of Daily Living (ADL) index score following stroke. *Clin Rehabil.* 1998;12(4):277-280.

Tsubokawa T, Katayama Y, Yamamoto T. Control of persistent hemiballismus by chronic thalamic stimulation. Report of two cases. *J Neurosurg.* 1995;82(3):501-505.

Visocchi M, et al. Increase of cerebral blood flow and improvement of brain motor control following spinal cord stimulation in ischemic spastic hemiparesis. *Stereotact Funct Neurosurg.* 1994;62(1-4):103-107.

Wang RY, Tsai MW, Chan RC. Effects of surface spinal cord stimulation on spasticity and quantitative assessment of muscle tone in hemiplegic patients. *Am J Phys Med Rehabil.* 1998;77(4):282-287.

Weingarden HP, et al. Hybrid functional electrical stimulation orthosis system for the upper limb: effects on spasticity in chronic stable hemiplegia. *Am J Phys Med Rehabil.* 1998;77(4):276-281.

Electrotherapeutic Terminology in Physical Therapy

Wong AM, et al. Clinical trial of electrical acupuncture on hemiplegic stroke patients. *Am J Phys Med Rehabil.* 1999;78(2):117-122.

Zhang X, et al. The changes of vasoactive intestinal peptide somatostatin and pancreatic polypeptide in blood and CSF of acute cerebral infarction patients and the effect of acupuncture on them [in Chinese]. *Chen Tzu Yen Chiu.* 1996;21(4):10-16.

Peripheral Nervous System (PNS)

Chang CW, Lien IN. Tardy effect of neurogenic muscular atrophy by magnetic stimulation. *Am J Phys Med Rehabil.* 1994;73(4):275-279.

Clemente FR, Barron KW. Transcutaneous neuromuscular electrical stimulation effect on the degree of microvascular perfusion in autonomically denervated rat skeletal muscle. *Arch Phys Med Rehabil.* 1996;77(2):155-160.

Eberstein A, Eberstein S. Electrical stimulation of denervated muscle: is it worthwhile? *Med Sci Sports Exerc.* 1996;28(12):1463-1469.

Farragher D, Kidd GL, Tallis R. Eutrophic electrical stimulation for Bell's palsy. *Clin Rehabil.* 1987;1:265-271.

Gittins J, et al. Electrical stimulation as a therapeutic option to improve eyelid function in chronic facial nerve disorders. *Invest Ophthalmol Vis Sci.* 1999;40(3):547-554.

Hussain SS, Winterburn SJ, Grace AR. Eutrophic electrical stimulation in long-standing facial palsy. *Eur Arch Otorhinolaryngol Suppl.* 1994;S133-134.

Kanaya F, Tajima T. Effect of electrostimulation on denervated muscle. *Clin Orthop.* 1992;(283):296-301.

Kern H, et al. Standing up with denervated muscles in humans using functional electrical stimulation. *Artif Organs.* 1999;23(5):447-452.

Mokrusch T, et al. Effects of long-impulse electrical stimulation on atrophy and fibre type composition of chronically denervated fast rabbit muscle. *J Neurol.* 1990;237(1):29-34.

Neumayer C, et al. Hypertrophy and transformation of muscle fibers in paraplegic patients. *Artif Organs.* 1997;21(3):188-190.

Nix WA, Dahm M. The effect of isometric short-term electrical stimulation on denervated muscle. *Muscle Nerve.* 1987;10(2):136-143.

Reichel M, Mayr W, Rattay F. Computer simulation of field distribution and excitation of denervated muscle fibers caused by surface electrodes. *Artif Organs.* 1999;23(5):453-456.

Rothstein J, Berlinger NT. Electronic reanimation of facial paralysis: a feasibility study. *Otolaryngol Head Neck Surg.* 1986;94(1):82-85.

Salerno GM, Bleicher JN, McBride DM. Restoration of paralyzed orbicularis oculi muscle function by controlled electrical current. *J Invest Surg.* 1991;4(4):445-456.

Stennert E, et al. Effects of electrostimulation therapie: enzyme-histological and myometric changes in the denervated musculature. *Eur Arch Otorhinolaryngol Suppl.* 1994;S37-41.

Stief CG, et al. Functional electromyostimulation of the corpus cavernosum penis: preliminary results of a novel therapeutic option for erectile dysfunction. *World J Urol.* 1995;13(4):243-247.

Targan RS, Alon G, Kay SL. Effect of long-term electrical stimulation on motor recovery and improvement of clinical residuals in patients with unresolved facial nerve palsy. *Otolaryngol Head Neck Surg.* 2000;122(2):246-252.

Valencic V, et al. Improved motor response due to chronic electrical stimulation of denervated tibialis anterior muscle in humans. *Muscle Nerve.* 1986;9(7):612-617.

Williams HB. A clinical pilot study to assess functional return following continuous muscle stimulation after nerve injury and repair in the upper extremity using a completely implantable electrical system. *Microsurgery.* 1996;17(11):597-605.

Woodcock AH, Taylor PN, Ewins DJ. Long pulse biphasic electrical stimulation of denervated muscle. *Artif Organs.* 1999;23(5):457-459.

Primary Muscular Dystrophy (PMD)

Dangain J, Vrbova G. Long term effect of low frequency chronic electrical stimulation on the fast hind limb muscles of dystrophic mice. *J Neurol Neurosurg Psychiatry.* 1989;52(12):1382-1389.

Dubowitz V. Responses of diseased muscle to electrical and mechanical intervention. *Ciba Found Symp.* 1988;138:240-255.

Edwards RH, et al. Practical analysis of variability of muscle function measurements in Duchenne muscular dystrophy. *Muscle Nerve.* 1987;10(1):6-14.

Scott OM, et al. Responses of muscles of patients with Duchenne muscular dystrophy to chronic electrical stimulation. *J Neurol Neurosurg Psychiatry.* 1986;49(12):1427-1434.

Scott OM, et al. Therapeutic possibilities of chronic low frequency electrical stimulation in children with Duchenne muscular dystrophy. *J Neurol Sci.* 1990;95(2):171-182.

Yoshida M, et al. Skeletal muscle fiber degeneration in mdx mice induced by electrical stimulation. *Muscle Nerve.* 1997;20(11):1422-1432.

Zupan A, et al. Effects of electrical stimulation on muscles of children with Duchenne and Becker muscular dystrophy. *Neuropediatrics.* 1993;24(4):189-192.

Zupan A. Long-term electrical stimulation of muscles in children with Duchenne and Becker muscular dystrophy. *Muscle Nerve.* 1992;15(3):362-367.

Joint Mobility

Anderson AF, Lipscomb AB. Analysis of rehabilitation techniques after anterior cruciate reconstruction. *Am J Sports Med.* 1989;17(2):154-160.

Gotlin RS, et al. Electrical stimulation effect on extensor lag and length of hospital stay after total knee arthroplasty. *Arch Phys Med Rehabil.* 1994;75(9):957-959.

Jensen JE, et al. The use of transcutaneous neural stimulation and isokinetic testing in arthroscopic knee surgery. *Am J Sports Med.* 1985;13(1):27-33.

Linde C, Isacsson G, Jonsson BG. Outcome of 6-week treatment with transcutaneous electric nerve stimulation compared with splint on symptomatic temporomandibular joint disk displacement without reduction. *Acta Odontol Scand.* 1995;53(2):92-98.

McCaffery M,. Wolff M. Pain relief using cutaneous modalities, positioning, and movement. *Hosp J.* 1992;8(1-2):121-153.

Melzack R, Vetere R, Finch L. Transcutaneous electrical nerve stimulation for low back pain. A comparison of TENS and massage for pain and range of motion. *Phys Ther.* 1983;63(4):489-493.

Morgan B, et al. Transcutaneous electric nerve stimulation (TENS) during distension shoulder arthrography: a controlled trial. *Pain.* 1996;64(2):265-267.

Pope MH, et al. A prospective randomized three-week trial of spinal manipulation, transcutaneous muscle stimulation, massage and corset in the treatment of subacute low back pain. *Spine.* 1994;19(22):2571-2577.

Rizk TE, et al. Adhesive capsulitis (frozen shoulder): a new approach to its management. *Arch Phys Med Rehabil.* 1983;64(1):29-33.

Rizk TE, Park SJ. Transcutaneous electrical nerve stimulation and extensor splint in linear scleroderma knee contracture. *Arch Phys Med Rehabil.* 1981;62(2):86-88.

Walker RH, et al. Postoperative use of continuous passive motion, transcutaneous electrical nerve stimulation, and continuous cooling pad following total knee arthroplasty. *J Arthroplasty.* 1991;6(2):151-156.

Werner S, et al. Electrical stimulation of vastus medialis and stretching of lateral thigh muscles in patients with patello-femoral symptoms. *Knee Surg Sports Traumatol Arthrosc.* 1993;1(2):85-92.

Zizic TM, et al. The treatment of osteoarthritis of the knee with pulsed electrical stimulation. *J Rheumatol.* 1995;22(9):1757-1761.

Tissue Repair

Agren MS, Engel MA, Mertz PM. Collagenase during burn wound healing: influence of a hydrogel dressing and pulsed electrical stimulation. *Plast Reconstr Surg.* 1994;94(3):518-524.

Baker LL, et al. Effects of electrical stimulation on wound healing in patients with diabetic ulcers. *Diabetes Care.* 1997;20(3):405-412.

Carley PJ, Wainapel SF. Electrotherapy for acceleration of wound healing: low intensity direct current. *Arch Phys Med Rehabil.* 1985;66(7):443-446.

Cosmo P, et al. Effects of transcutaneous nerve stimulation on the microcirculation in chronic leg ulcers. *Scand J Plast Reconstr Surg Hand Surg.* 2000;34(1):61-64.

Davis SC, Ovington LG. Electrical stimulation and ultrasound in wound healing. *Dermatol Clin.* 1993;11(4):775-781.

Feedar JA, Kloth LC, Gentzkow GD. Chronic dermal ulcer healing enhanced with monophasic pulsed electrical stimulation [see comment in *Phys Ther.* 1992;72(7):539]. *Phys Ther.* 1991;71(9):639-649.

Finsen V, et al. Transcutaneous electrical nerve stimulation after major amputation. *J Bone Joint Surg Br.* 1988;70(1):109-112.

Fitzgerald GK, Newsome D. Treatment of a large infected thoracic spine wound using high voltage pulsed monophasic current. *Phys Ther.* 1993;73(6):355-360.

Frantz RA, et al. Adoption of research-based practice for treatment of pressure ulcers in long-term care. *Decubitus.* 1992;5(1):44-45, 48-54.

Gardner SE, Frantz RA, Schmidt FL. Effect of electrical stimulation on chronic wound healing: a meta-analysis. *Wound Repair Regen.* 1999;7(6):495-503.

Gentzkow GD, et al. Healing of refractory stage III and IV pressure ulcers by a new electrical stimulation device. *Wounds.* 1993;5:160-172.

Gilcreast DM, et al. Effect of electrical stimulation on foot skin perfusion in persons with or at risk for diabetic foot ulcers. *Wound Repair Regen.* 1998;6(5):434-441.

Gogia PP, Marquez RR, Minerbo GM. Effects of high voltage galvanic stimulation on wound healing. *Ostomy Wound Manage.* 1992;38(1):29-35.

Griffin JW, et al. Efficacy of high voltage pulsed current for healing of pressure ulcers in patients with spinal cord injury. *Phys Ther.* 1991;71(6):433-442; discussion 442-444.

Hafner J. Management of arterial leg ulcers and of combined (mixed) venous-arterial leg ulcers. *Curr Probl Dermatol.* 1999;27:211-219.

Junger M, et al. Treatment of venous ulcers with low frequency pulsed current (Dermapulse): effects on cutaneous microcirculation [in German]. *Hautarzt.* 1997;48(12):897-903.

Kaada B, Emru M. Promoted healing of leprous ulcers by transcutaneous nerve stimulation. *Acupunct Electrother Res.* 1988;13(4):165-176.

Kloth LC, Feedar JA. Acceleration of wound healing with high voltage, monophasic, pulsed current [see erratum in *Phys Ther.* 1989;69(8):702]. *Phys Ther.* 1988;68(4):503-508.

Kloth LC, McCulloch JM. Promotion of wound healing with electrical stimulation. *Adv Wound Care.* 1996;9(5):42-45.

Lundeberg T, Kjartansson J, Samuelsson U. Effect of electrical nerve stimulation on healing of ischaemic skin flaps. *Lancet.* 1988;2(8613):712-714.

Lundeberg TC, Eriksson SV, Malm M. Electrical nerve stimulation improves healing of diabetic ulcers. *Ann Plast Surg.* 1992;29(4):328-331.

Mawson AR, et al. Effect of high voltage pulsed galvanic stimulation on sacral transcutaneous oxygen tension levels in the spinal cord injured. *Paraplegia.* 1993;31(5):311-319.

Mulder GD, Treatment of open-skin wounds with electric stimulation [see comment in *Phys Ther.* 1991;72(6):375-377]. *Arch Phys Med Rehabil.* 1991;72(6):375-377.

Politis MJ, Zanakis MF, Miller JE. Enhanced survival of full-thickness skin grafts following the application of DC electrical fields. *Plast Reconstr Surg.* 1989;84(2):267-272.

Prentice D, Theriault K. Clinical comment on the Dermapulse Wound Management System [corrected] [published erratum appears in *Perspectives* 1995;19(4):24]. *Perspectives.* 1995;19(3):7-8.

Stefanovska A, et al. Treatment of chronic wounds by means of electric and electromagnetic fields, II: value of FES parameters for pressure sore treatment. *Med Biol Eng Comput.* 1993;31(3):213-220.

Stromberg BV. Effects of electrical currents on wound contraction. *Ann Plast Surg.* 1988;21(2):121-123.

Sumano H, Mateos G. The use of acupuncture-like electrical stimulation for wound healing of lesions unresponsive to conventional treatment. *Am J Acupunct.* 1999;27(1-2):5-14.

Unger PG. Wound healing currents: a brief review of recent research points to electrical stimulation as a viable treatment technique. *Rehab Manag.* 1992;5(3):42-43.

Weiss DS, Eaglstein WH, Falanga V. Exogenous electric current can reduce the formation of hypertrophic scars. *J Dermatol Surg Oncol.* 1989;15(12):1272-1275.

Wood JM, et al. A multicenter study on the use of pulsed low-intensity direct current for healing chronic stage II and stage III decubitus ulcers [see comment in *Arch Dermatol.* 1994;130(5):660-661]. *Arch Dermatol.* 1993;129(8):999-1009.

Acute and Chronic Edema

Bettany JA, Fish DR, Mendel FC. High-voltage pulsed direct current: effect on edema formation after hyperflexion injury. *Arch Phys Med Rehabil.* 1990;71(9):677-681.

Bettany JA, Fish DR, Mendel FC. Influence of high voltage pulsed direct current on edema formation following impact injury [see comment in *Phys Ther.* 1990;70(9):583-586]. *Phys Ther.* 1990;70(4):219-224.

Chu CS, et al. Direct current reduces accumulation of Evans Blue albumin in full- thickness burns. *J Trauma.* 1999;47(2):294-299.

Chu CS, et al. Direct current reduces wound edema after full-thickness burn injury in rats. *J Trauma.* 1996;40(5):738-742.

Cook HA, et al. Effects of electrical stimulation on lymphatic flow and limb volume in the rat. *Phys Ther.* 1994;74(11):1040-1046.

Cosgrove KA, et al. The electrical effect of two commonly used clinical stimulators on traumatic edema in rats. *Phys Ther.* 1992;72(3):227-233.

Faghri PD, et al. Electrical stimulation-induced contraction to reduce blood stasis during arthroplasty. *IEEE Trans Rehabil Eng.* 1997;5(1):62-69.

Faghri PD. The effects of neuromuscular stimulation-induced muscle contraction versus elevation on hand edema in CVA patients. *J Hand Ther.* 1997;10(1):29-34.

Fish DR, et al. Effect of anodal high voltage pulsed current on edema formation in frog hind limbs. *Phys Ther.* 1991;71(10):724-730; discussion 730-733.

Gerasimenko VN, Grushina TI, Lev SG. A complex of conservative rehabilitation measures in postmastectomy edema [in Russian]. *Vopr Onkol.* 1990;36(12):1479-1485.

Gonzalez-Darder J, Canadas-Rodriguez D. Effects of cervical spinal cord stimulation in experimental ischaemic oedema. *Neurol Res.* 1991;13(4):229-232.

Griffin JW, et al. Reduction of chronic posttraumatic hand edema: a comparison of high voltage pulsed current, intermittent pneumatic compression, and placebo treatments. *Phys Ther.* 1990;70(5):279-286.

Karnes JL, et al. High-voltage pulsed current: its influence on diameters of histamine- dilated arterioles in hamster cheek pouches. *Arch Phys Med Rehabil.* 1995;76(4):381-386.

Karnes JL, Mendel FC, Fish DR, Effects of low voltage pulsed current on edema formation in frog hind limbs following impact injury. *Phys Ther.* 1992;72(4):273-278.

Lanham RH Jr, Powell S, Hendrix BE. Efficacy of hypothermia and transcutaneous electrical nerve stimulation in podiatric surgery. *J Foot Surg.* 1984;23(2):152-158.

Mendel FC, Wylegala JA, Fish DR, Influence of high voltage pulsed current on edema formation following impact injury in rats. *Phys Ther.* 1992;72(9):668-673.

Michlovitz S, Smith W, and Watkins, M. Ice and high voltage pulsed stimulation in treatment of lateral ankle sprains. *Orthop Sports Phys Ther.* 1988;9:301-304.

Mir LM, et al. Systemic antitumor effects of electrochemotherapy combined with histoincompatible cells secreting interleukin-2. *J Immunother Emphasis Tumor Immunol.* 1995;17(1):30-38.

Mohr TM, Akers TK, Landry RG. Effect of high voltage stimulation on edema reduction in the rat hind limb. *Phys Ther.* 1987;67(11):1703-1707.

Paris DL, Baynes F, Gucker B. Effects of the neuroprobe in the treatment of second-degree ankle inversion sprains. *Phys Ther.* 1983;63(1):35-40.

Ross CR, Sega D. High voltage galvanic stimulation-an aid to post-operative healing. *Curr Podiatry.* 1981;30:19-25.

Stralka SW, Jackson JA, Lewis AR. Treatment of hand and wrist pain: a randomized clinical trial of high voltage pulsed, direct current built into a wrist splint. *Aaohn J.* 1998;46(5):233-236.

Taylor K, et al. Effect of a single 30-minute treatment of high voltage pulsed current on edema formation in frog hind limbs. *Phys Ther.* 1992;72(1):63-68.

Thornton RM, Mendel FC, Fish DR. Effects of electrical stimulation on edema formation in different strains of rats. *Phys Ther.* 1998;78(4):386-394.

Voight ML. Reduction of post-traumatic ankle edema with high voltage pulsed galvanic stimulation. *Athletic Training.* 1984;19:278-279.

Weinberger A, et al. Transcutaneous electrical stimulation of the normal rabbit joint. *Scand J Rehabil Med.* 1987;19(2):67-70.

Wojtys EM, Carpenter JE, Ott GA. Electrical stimulation of soft tissues. *Instr Course Lect.* 1993;42:443-452.

Peripheral Circulation Impairments

Badylak SF, et al. The effect of skeletal muscle ventricle pouch pressure on muscle blood flow. *Asaio J.* 1992;38(1):66-71.

Balogun JA, Biasci S, Han L. The effects of acupuncture, electroneedling and transcutaneous electrical stimulation therapies on peripheral haemodynamic functioning [see comments in Disabil Rehabil. 1999;21(3):129-130, 133, 134-136; discussion 137-138]. *Disabil Rehabil.* 1998;20(2):41-48.

Bjorna H, Kaada B. Successful treatment of itching and atopic eczema by transcutaneous nerve stimulation. *Acupunct Electrother Res.* 1987;12(2):101-112.

Bodenheim R, Bennett JH. Reversal of a Sudeck's atrophy by the adjunctive use of transcutaneous electrical nerve stimulation: a case report. *Phys Ther.* 1983;63(8):1287-1288.

Cook HA, et al. Effects of electrical stimulation on lymphatic flow and limb volume in the rat. *Phys Ther.* 1994;74(11):1040-1046.

Cooney WP. Electrical stimulation and the treatment of complex regional pain syndromes of the upper extremity. *Hand Clin.* 1997;13(3):519-526.

Cosmo P, et al. Effects of transcutaneous nerve stimulation on the microcirculation in chronic leg ulcers. *Scand J Plast Reconstr Surg Hand Surg.* 2000;34(1):61-64.

Cramp AF, et al. The effect of high- and low-frequency transcutaneous electrical nerve stimulation upon cutaneous blood flow and skin temperature in healthy subjects. *Clin Physiol.* 2000;20(2):150-157.

Debreceni L, et al. Results of transcutaneous electrical stimulation (TES) in cure of lower extremity arterial disease. *Angiology.* 1995;46(7):613-618.

Faghri PD, et al. Electrical stimulation-induced contraction to reduce blood stasis during arthroplasty. *IEEE Trans Rehabil Eng.* 1997;5(1):62-69.

Faghri PD, Votto JJ, Hovorka CF. Venous hemodynamics of the lower extremities in response to electrical stimulation. *Arch Phys Med Rehabil.* 1998;79(7):842-848.

Forster RS, Fu FH. Reflex sympathetic dystrophy in children. A case report and review of literature. *Orthopedics.* 1985;8(4):475-477.

Gobelet C, et al. Calcitonin and reflex sympathetic dystrophy syndrome. *Clin Rheumatol.* 1986;5(3):382-388.

Hareau J. What makes treatment for reflex sympathetic dystrophy successful? *J Hand Ther.* 1996;9(4):367-370.

Heath ME, Gibbs SB. High-voltage pulsed galvanic stimulation: effects of frequency of current on blood flow in the human calf muscle. *Clin Sci (Colch).* 1992;82(6):607-613.

Junger M, et al. Treatment of venous ulcers with low frequency pulsed current (Dermapulse): effects on cutaneous microcirculation [in German]. *Hautarzt.* 1997;48(12):897-903.

Kaada B, Emru M. Promoted healing of leprous ulcers by transcutaneous nerve stimulation. *Acupunct Electrother Res.* 1988;13(4):165-176.

Kaada B, et al. Transcutaneous nerve stimulation in patients with coronary arterial disease: haemodynamic and biochemical effects. *Eur Heart J.* 1990;11(5):447-453.

Kaada B, Hognestad S, Havstad J. Transcutaneous nerve stimulation (TNS) in tinnitus. *Scand Audiol.* 1989;18(4):211-217.

Kaada B, Lygren I. Lower plasma levels of some gastrointestinal peptides in Raynaud's disease: influence of transcutaneous nerve stimulation. *Gen Pharmacol.* 1985;16(2):153-156.

Kaada B. Improvement of physical performance by transcutaneous nerve stimulation in athletes. *Acupunct Electrother Res.* 1984;9(3):165-180.

Kaada B. Successful treatment of esophageal dysmotility and Raynaud's phenomenon in systemic sclerosis and achalasia by transcutaneous nerve stimulation: increase in plasma VIP concentration. Scand *J Gastroenterol.* 1987;22(9):1137-1146.

Kaada B. Systemic sclerosis: successful treatment of ulcerations, pain, Raynaud's phenomenon, calcinosis, and dysphagia by transcutaneous nerve stimulation—a case report. *Acupunct Electrother Res.* 1984;9(1):31-44.

Kaada B. Treatment of fibromyalgia by low-frequency transcutaneous nerve stimulation [in Norwegian]. *Tidsskr Nor Laegeforen.* 1989;109(29):2992-2995.

Kaada B. Vasodilation induced by transcutaneous nerve stimulation in peripheral ischemia: (Raynaud's phenomenon and diabetic polyneuropathy). *Eur Heart J.* 1982;3(4):303-314.

Kao W, et al. Abnormalities of skeletal muscle metabolism during nerve stimulation determined by 31P nuclear magnetic resonance spectroscopy in severe congestive heart failure. *Am J Cardiol.* 1995;76(8):606-609.

Karnes JL, et al. High-voltage pulsed current: its influence on diameters of histamine- dilated arterioles in hamster cheek pouches. *Arch Phys Med Rehabil.* 1995;76(4):381-386.

Katz RT, et al. Functional electric stimulation to enhance systemic fibrinolytic activity in spinal cord injury patients. *Arch Phys Med Rehabil.* 1987;68(7):423-426.

Kesler RW, et al. Reflex sympathetic dystrophy in children: treatment with transcutaneous electric nerve stimulation. *Pediatrics.* 1988;82(5):728-732.

Klecker N, Theiss W. Transcutaneous electric muscle stimulation: a "new" possibility for the prevention of thrombosis? [in German]. *Vasa.* 1994;23(1):23-29.

Kruk M, et al. Rheographic evaluation of the changes in blood flow after superficial electric stimulation in patients with Raynaud's disease or syndrome [in Polish]. *Pol Tyg Lek.* 1989;44(43-45):921-923.

Leo KC. Use of electrical stimulation at acupuncture points for the treatment of reflex sympathetic dystrophy in a child: a case report. *Phys Ther.* 1983;63(6):957-959.

Lindstrom B, et al. Electrically induced short-lasting tetanus of the calf muscles for prevention of deep vein thrombosis. *Br J Surg.* 1982;69(4):203-206.

Loubser PG, et al. Effects of unilateral, low-frequency, neuromuscular stimulation on superficial circulation in lower extremities of patients with peripheral vascular disease. *Med Instrum.* 1988;22(2):82-87.

Maillefert JF, et al. Effects of low-frequency electrical stimulation of quadriceps and calf muscles in patients with chronic heart failure. *J Cardiopulm Rehabil.* 1998;18(4):277-282.

Miller BF, Gruben KG, Morgan BJ. Circulatory responses to voluntary and electrically induced muscle contractions in humans. *Phys Ther.* 2000;80(1):53-60.

Mulder P, et al. Transcutaneous electrical nerve stimulation (TENS) in Raynaud's phenomenon. *Angiology.* 1991;42(5):414-417.

Peters EJ, et al. The benefit of electrical stimulation to enhance perfusion in persons with diabetes mellitus. *J Foot Ankle Surg.* 1998;37(5):396-400; discussion 447-448.

Quittan M, et al. Strength improvement of knee extensor muscles in patients with chronic heart failure by neuromuscular electrical stimulation. *Artif Organs.* 1999;23(5):432-435.

Robaina FJ, et al. Transcutaneous electrical nerve stimulation and spinal cord stimulation for pain relief in reflex sympathetic dystrophy. *Stereotact Funct Neurosurg.* 1989;52(1):53-62.

Sanderson JE, et al. The effect of transcutaneous electrical nerve stimulation (TENS) on autonomic cardiovascular reflexes. *Clin Auton Res.* 1995;5(2):81-84.

Wikstrom SO, et al. Effect of transcutaneous nerve stimulation on microcirculation in intact skin and blister wounds in healthy volunteers. *Scand J Plast Reconstr Surg Hand Surg.* 1999;33(2):195-201.

Wilder RT, et al. Reflex sympathetic dystrophy in children: clinical characteristics and follow-up of seventy patients. *J Bone Joint Surg Am.* 1992;74(6):910-919.

Incontinence

Appell RA. Electrical stimulation for the treatment of urinary incontinence. *Urology.* 1998;51(2A Suppl):24-26.

Aristizabal Agudelo JM, et al. Urodynamic results of the treatment of urinary incontinence with peripheral electric stimulation [in Spanish]. *Arch Esp Urol.* 1996;49(8):836-842.

Balcom AH, et al. Initial experience with home therapeutic electrical stimulation for continence in the myelomeningocele population. *J Urol.* 1997;158(3 Pt 2):1272-1276.

Berghmans LC, et al. Conservative treatment of stress urinary incontinence in women: a systematic review of randomized clinical trials. *Br J Urol.* 1998;82(2):181-191.

Bo K, Maanum M. Does vaginal electrical stimulation cause pelvic floor muscle contraction?: a pilot study. *Scand J Urol Nephrol Suppl.* 1996;179:39-45.

Bo K, Talseth T, Holme I. Single blind, randomised controlled trial of pelvic floor exercises, electrical stimulation, vaginal cones, and no treatment in management of genuine stress incontinence in women. *Bmj.* 1999;318(7182):487-493.

Bo K. Effect of electrical stimulation on stress and urge urinary incontinence: clinical outcome and practical recommendations based on randomized controlled trials. *Acta Obstet Gynecol Scand Suppl.* 1998;168:3-11.

Bower WF, et al. A urodynamic study of surface neuromodulation versus sham in detrusor instability and sensory urgency. *J Urol.* 1998;160(6 Pt 1):2133-2136.

Bratt H, et al. Long-term effects ten years after maximal electrostimulation of the pelvic floor in women with unstable detrusor and urge incontinence. *Acta Obstet Gynecol Scand Suppl.* 1998;168:22-24.

Brubaker L, et al. Transvaginal electrical stimulation for female urinary incontinence. *Am J Obstet Gynecol.* 1997;177(3):536-540.

Dumoulin C, et al. Pelvic-floor rehabilitation, I: Comparison of two surface electrode placements during stimulation of the pelvic-floor musculature in women who are continent using bipolar interferential currents. *Phys Ther.* 1995;75(12):1067-1074.

Esa A, et al. Functional electrical stimulation in the management of incontinence: studies of urodynamics. *Int Urol Nephrol.* 1991;23(2):135-141.

Fall M, Lindstrom S. Electrical stimulation: a physiologic approach to the treatment of urinary incontinence. *Urol Clin North Am.* 1991;18(2):393-407.

Fall M. Advantages and pitfalls of functional electrical stimulation. *Acta Obstet Gynecol Scand Suppl.* 1998;168:16-21.

Geirsson G, Fall M. Maximal functional electrical stimulation in routine practice. *Neurourol Urodyn.* 1997;16(6):559-565.

Jonasson A, et al. Short-term maximal electrical stimulation: a conservative treatment of urinary incontinence. *Gynecol Obstet Invest.* 1990;30(2):120-123.

Kontani H, Hayashi K. Urinary bladder response to hypogastric nerve stimulation after bilateral resection of the pelvic nerve or spinal cord injury in rats. *Int J Urol.* 1997;4(4):394-400.

Kralj B. Conservative treatment of female stress urinary incontinence with functional electrical stimulation. *Eur J Obstet Gynecol Reprod Biol.* 1999;85(1):53-56.

Kulseng-Hanssen S, Kristoffersen M, Larsen E. Evaluation of the subjective and objective effect of maximal electrical stimulation in patients complaining of urge incontinence. *Acta Obstet Gynecol Scand Suppl.* 1998;168:12-15.

Luber KM, Wolde-Tsadik G. Efficacy of functional electrical stimulation in treating genuine stress incontinence: a randomized clinical trial. *Neurourol Urodyn.* 1997;16(6):543-551.

Malissard M, Souquet J, Jullien D. Optimisation of pulse duration for intravaginal electrical stimulation: effect of tissue excitability. *Med Biol Eng Comput.* 1994;32(3):327-330.

Marshall DF, Boston VE. Altered bladder and bowel function following cutaneous electrical field stimulation in children with spina bifida: interim results of a randomized double-blind placebo-controlled trial. *Eur J Pediatr Surg.* 1997;7 Suppl 1:41-43.

Meyer S, et al. Subjective and objective effects of intravaginal electrical myostimulation and biofeedback in patients with genuine stress urinary incontinence. *Br J Urol.* 1992;69(6):584-588.

Miller K, et al. Pelvic floor electrical stimulation for genuine stress incontinence: who will benefit and when? *Int Urogynecol J Pelvic Floor Dysfunct.* 1998;9(5):265-270.

Moore KN. Treatment of urinary incontinence in men with electrical stimulation: is practice evidence-based? *J Wound Ostomy Continence Nurs.* 2000;27(1):20-31.

Moul JW. Pelvic muscle rehabilitation in males following prostatectomy. *Urol Nurs.* 1998;18(4):296-301.

Okada N, et al. Transcutaneous electrical stimulation of thigh muscles in the treatment of detrusor overactivity. *Br J Urol.* 1998;81(4):560-564.

Primus G, Kramer G. Maximal external electrical stimulation for treatment of neurogenic or non-neurogenic urgency and/or urge incontinence. *Neurourol Urodyn.* 1996;15(3):187-194.

Primus G. Maximal electrical stimulation in neurogenic detrusor hyperactivity: experiences in multiple sclerosis. *Eur J Med.* 1992;1(2):80-82.

Richardson DA, et al. Pelvic floor electrical stimulation: a comparison of daily and every-other-day therapy for genuine stress incontinence. *Urology.* 1996;48(1):110-118.

Sand PK, et al. Pelvic floor electrical stimulation in the treatment of genuine stress incontinence: a multi-center, placebo-controlled trial. *Am J Obstet Gynecol.* 1995;173(1):72-79.

Seim A, Hermstad R, Hunskaar S. Female urinary incontinence: long-term follow-up after treatment in general practice [see comment in *Br J Gen Pract.* 1998;48(436):1727-1728]. *Br J Gen Pract.* 1998;48(436):1731-1734.

Siegel SW, et al. Pelvic floor electrical stimulation for the treatment of urge and mixed urinary incontinence in women. *Urology.* 1997;50(6):934-940.

Smith JJ 3rd. Intravaginal stimulation randomized trial. *J Urol.* 1996;155(1):127-130.

Sung MS, et al. The effect of pelvic floor muscle exercises on genuine stress incontinence among Korean women: focusing on its effects on the quality of life. *Yonsei Med J.* 2000;41(2):237-251.

Trsinar B, Kraij B. Maximal electrical stimulation in children with unstable bladder and nocturnal enuresis and/or daytime incontinence: a controlled study. *Neurourol Urodyn.* 1996;15(2):133-142.

Vahtera T, et al. Pelvic floor rehabilitation is effective in patients with multiple sclerosis. *Clin Rehabil.* 1997;11(3):211-219.

Yamanishi T, et al. Pelvic floor electrical stimulation in the treatment of stress incontinence: an investigational study and a placebo controlled double-blind trial. *J Urol.* 1997;158(6):2127-2131.

Yamanishi T, et al. Randomized, double-blind study of electrical stimulation for urinary incontinence due to detrusor overactivity. *Urology.* 2000;55(3):353-357.

Yokoyama O, et al. Experimental and clinical evaluation of functional electrical stimulation of the anal sphincter [in Japanese]. *Hinyokika Kiyo.* 1992;38(10):1109-1115.

Zollner-Nielsen M, Samuelsson SM. Maximal electrical stimulation of patients with frequency, urgency and urge incontinence: report of 38 cases. *Acta Obstet Gynecol Scand.* 1992;71(8):629-631.

Iontophoresis

Banta CA. A prospective, nonrandomized study of iontophoresis, wrist splinting, and antiinflammatory medication in the treatment of early-mild carpal tunnel syndrome. *J Occup Med.* 1994;36(2):166-168.

Braun BL. Treatment of an acute anterior disk displacement in the temporomandibular joint: a case report. *Phys Ther.* 1987;67(8):1234-1236.

Chandler TJ. Iontophoresis of 0.4% dexamethasone for plantar fasciitis. *Clin J Sport Med.* 1998;8(1):68.

Chantraine A, Ludy JP, Berger D. Is cortisone iontophoresis possible? *Arch Phys Med Rehabil.* 1986;67(1):38-40.

Gangarosa LP Sr, et al. Iontophoresis for enhancing penetration of dermatologic and antiviral drugs. *J Dermatol.* 1995;22(11):865-875.

Garza HH Jr, Hill JM. Effect of a beta-adrenergic antagonist, propranolol, on induced HSV-1 ocular recurrence in latently infected rabbits. *Curr Eye Res.* 1997;16(5):453-458.

Gudeman SD, et al. Treatment of plantar fasciitis by iontophoresis of 0.4% dexamethasone. A randomized, double-blind, placebo-controlled study. *Am J Sports Med.* 1997;25(3):312-316.

Hasson SM, et al. Dexamethasone iontophoresis: effect on delayed muscle soreness and muscle function [see comment in *Can J Sport Sci.* 1992;17(1):74]. *Can J Sport Sci.* 1992;17(1):8-13.

Howard JP, Drake TR, Kellogg DL Jr. Effects of alternating current iontophoresis on drug delivery. *Arch Phys Med Rehabil.* 1995;76(5):463-466.

Kamath SS, Gangarosa LP Sr, Electrophoretic evaluation of the mobility of drugs suitable for iontophoresis. *Methods Find Exp Clin Pharmacol.* 1995;17(4):227-232.

Lam TT, et al. Transscleral iontophoresis of dexamethasone. *Arch Ophthalmol.* 1989;107(9):1368-1371.

Li LC, et al. The efficacy of dexamethasone iontophoresis for the treatment of rheumatoid arthritic knees: a pilot study. *Arthritis Care Res.* 1996;9(2):126-132.

Montorsi F, et al. Transdermal electromotive multi-drug administration for Peyronie's disease: preliminary results. *J Androl.* 2000;21(1):85-90.

Reid KI, et al. Evaluation of iontophoretically applied dexamethasone for painful pathologic temporomandibular joints. *Oral Surg Oral Med Oral Pathol.* 1994;77(6):605-609.

Riedl CR, et al. Intravesical electromotive drug administration technique: preliminary results and side effects. *J Urol.* 1998;159(6):1851-1856.

Riedl CR, et al. Iontophoresis for treatment of Peyronie's disease. *J Urol.* 2000;163(1):95-99.

Rosamilia A, Dwyer PL, Gibson J. Electromotive drug administration of lidocaine and dexamethasone followed by cystodistension in women with interstitial cystitis. *Int Urogynecol J Pelvic Floor Dysfunct.* 1997;8(3):142-145.

Sato H, Takahashi H, Honjo I. Transtympanic iontophoresis of dexamethasone and fosfomycin. *Arch Otolaryngol Head Neck Surg.* 1988;114(5):531-533.

Schiffman EL, Braun BL, Lindgren BR. Temporomandibular joint iontophoresis: a double-blind randomized clinical trial. *J Orofac Pain.* 1996;10(2):157-165.

Treffiletti S, et al. Iontophoresis in the conservative treatment of Peyronie's disease: preliminary experience [in Italian]. *Arch Ital Urol Androl.* 1997;69(5):323-327.

Verges J, Chateau A. New therapy for Peyronie's disease: superoxide dismutase by ionization [in French]. Comparison with an earlier classical series. *Ann Urol.* 1988;22(2):143-144.